Medicare Myths

by

Dennis J. Furlong M.D.

DREAMCATCHER PUBLISHING
Saint John • New Brunswick • Canada

DreamCatcher Publishing acknowledges the support of the New Brunswick Arts Council.

Canadian Cataloguing in Publication Data

Furlong, Dennis J. - 1945

Medicare Myths

ISBN - 1-894372-39-5
    1. Health care reform--Canada. 2. Medical policy--Canada. I. Title.
RA412.5.C3F87 2004   362.1'0971   C2004-902125-7

Editor: Yvonne Wilson

Typesetter: Chas Goguen

Cover Design: Dawn Drew, INK Graphic Design Services Corp.

Printed and bound in Canada

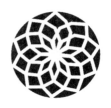

DREAMCATCHER PUBLISHING INC.
105 Prince William Street
Saint John, New Brunswick, Canada E2L 2B2
www.dreamcatcherbooks.ca

DEDICATION

This book is dedicated with love to my mom who is ninety-three years old and still pervades in a very positive way the existence of all of her seven children. She led by example and taught her children that every day is a good day, and every person is a good person.

ACKNOWLEDGEMENT

I would like to acknowledge and thank those who have encouraged and helped me in the production of this book:

Mr. Aubrey Browne	Toronto, ON
Mrs. Nicole Landry Bérubé	Dalhousie, NB
Mrs. Lisa Good	Charlo, NB
Mrs. Diane Hansen	Fredericton, NB
Mrs. Lynn Kelly de Groot	McLeods, NB
Mrs. Madelyn Doody	Halifax, NS

PREFACE

The Canadian Health Care System is currently in a quandary. It is clearly at a crossroad. It is consuming too much of Canada's financial resources now and continues to grow two or three times faster than any other government program, more or less out of control and to the detriment of all other government programs.

More aptly described, the Canadian Health Care System is at a fork in the road. Taking one fork is to continue the current system, continuing onward towards a financial impossibility. The other option is to take both forks: the first one being the public option cited above plus a second private system option; the second fork would lead us to a new separate private system for a few Canadian high-income earners, inconsistent with the Canadian mindset of egalitarianism.

My musings to follow show that we do not need to construct a new private system. We can think and act out of the proverbial box and make adjustments to solve the real problems in the present system and therefore retain it. We can make it a viable system that provides for Canadians' health care needs, not their wants.

My musings will undoubtedly not please some and I will be challenged, but it is colloquially, "time to call a spade a spade".

Certainly things that have not been said anywhere before but in the safety of corridor prattle now need to be said openly and publicly by all Canadians. I say "No to Romanow". Sorry, but his report is not the answer.

The Canadian people want to know if the system will be there for them in the future if they or their loved ones get "truly sick". I think it is possible to adjust the present system to make it sustainable.

Health care in Canada has been called a gorilla by politicians, especially by Premiers, Ministers of Finance and Ministers of Health, while they tear out their hair if they have any. My impression is that health care is indeed an aggressive unchained gorilla.

I think we are well able to re-cage and control the gorilla.

FOREWORD

Health reform is one of the greatest policy issues faced by this generation. The decisions literally will redefine Canadian Medicare. No wonder it has been the subject of discussion, commentary, articles and books, many of them authored by academics, economists and critics. Dr. Furlong brings a different view; one sculpted from his experience as the Minister of Health in New Brunswick and as a health practitioner. With his book, Dr. Furlong offers ideas that challenge both the status quo and how we think about it. Some of his ideas are new; some are controversial; all should be drawn upon to foster debate and explore all opportunities. We owe future generations of health care users nothing less.

Honourable Gary Mar
Minister of Health and Wellness
Province of Alberta

INTRODUCTION

The Canada Health Act is one of the most, if not the most, defining features of our country. Certainly it is the most defining feature of Canada's Health Care System.

We Canadians, in order to know ourselves better as Canadians, must see ourselves as others in the world see us. How then do others in the world see us? We rarely reflect on this as a people.

It has been constantly and repeatedly stated internationally for many years that Canada is one of the best countries in the world to live in. For the most part this is because of our wonderful social programs compared to the Americans' and other countries', and health care is indeed number one. Then **what is so terribly wrong with our public health system and the Canada Health Act if so many foreigners see it as such a pearl** and we see it as such a problem? It is my opinion that **not much is wrong.**

There is no doubt that the Canadian people see their publicly funded health care system as their most precious social program. It evolved from the initial efforts of Tommy Douglas in Saskatchewan forty-two years ago this year on July 2nd, 2004. It was to include coverage not only for hospital services but also for physicians' fees. Health services that were deemed medically necessary were to be insured, with a very loose definition of medically necessary. There was lots of money to go around and lots of political buy-in. Medically necessary meant 'all'. Then really, why all the acrimony?

In the early eighties under Federal Minister of Health Monique Bégin, the program was consolidated under the Canada Health Act, and extra billing by physicians was eliminated.

The Canada Health Act was passed in the House of Commons in a very unusual and almost unique and unprecedented way, unanimously! This was a clear indication of the universal popular support for the program.

The Canada Health Act had and still has five basic principles: To be accessible, portable, universal, publicly funded and comprehensive.

Accessibility simply means that hospital and physician services should be equally accessible to all Canadians. The challenge is of course that this is tempered by our great vast land mass.

Portability is defined as the privilege of having medically insured services anywhere in Canada, in any province, or in any territory, covered by the province of current residency.

Universality means that all Canadians are covered, again tempered by various residency rules such as living outside Canada in excess of a certain time period or interprovincial movement.

Publicly funded means that all health services defined as medically necessary are covered by tax based federal and provincial funding.

Comprehensive is the word initially used to attempt to describe the nature of what is medically necessary and therefore covered by the public purse.

The Canadian Health Care System remains the most valued, the most costly, the most criticized, the most abused, the most misused, the most overused public program, with funding shared between the federal government and its provincial and territorial partners.

Beyond all and any doubt and with the consideration of all factors, the Canadian Health Care System remains quite defensibly the best health care system in the world. All those who wish to tear it down in order to tear it up so to speak, for whatever personal or collective reasons, should be very concerned that they may get what they want. If one were to postulate a Canada without the Canadian publicly funded health care system, one could also postulate one in four Canadian physicians suddenly without work, along with another vast number of health providers and resultantly many patients unserved. Inevitably the best or the remaining doctors would have large accounts receivable and the usual problems of collection.

There have been several countries that "hit the fiscal wall" in their health care systems as a consequence of unlimited utilization and consumption of health care and no cost controls sagely applied to any of the three sides of the health care triangle. Sweden, England, the Netherlands, and New Zealand are some examples.

The health care triangle is the patient, the provider and the insurer. All these countries have gone straight into duality, or a public system and a separate parallel private system. Separate public and private health care systems in parallel, in Canada, may well not give Canadians 'better' health care. Better health care does not equal faster health care. Surely this change will not give improved wellness. In conversation with some Swedish, English and Dutch people they have related to me that many things are worse since duality, public and private.

Recently various individuals and groups have threatened to use the Canadian Charter of Rights to force the fracturing of the current health system into duality, into a public and a private system side by side. One must question how this is supposed to reduce and eliminate waiting lists for the general population. When one attempts to wrap this concept around one's neurons, the only conclusion possible is that it is paramountly ludicrous. There would unquestionably be marked benefits for a very few rich patients and marked benefits for a few providers who would no doubt become wealthier. The weakened public universal system would be inevitably more strained and would be for the rest, or the less-well-off population. The majority of common Canadians with health needs would therefore suffer further. Ironically, there would be much more damage to the health care system for the collective in the interest of the individual, resulting curiously in a poorer system for most individuals.

If, as Canadians, we do not make the correct decisions very soon in health care, and for the correct reasons, I believe that Canada will have lost something very good and unparalleled in our history. We will see the insatiable consumer demand for health care and the capitalistic wants and ambitions of some of the individual providers override the Canadian people's social benefits paid for by the collective tax base.

We Canadians made a decision some forty years ago to have a public system, a system that abandons no one and provides optimum egalitarian health care for all.

It is a system for the collective, the standards of which can only be decided by the collective.

The Americans call it socialism to demean its integrity. Ironically, patient behavior in the American fully-funded Medicade system for the poor is much like the behavior of Canadians in the Canadian Medicare system. Doctors who have worked in both voice this frequently. Medicade in America is completely free and often abused. Their private system coverage, however, has deductibles and is extremely expensive, fifty percent more per capita than in Canada as a percent of gross domestic product. It is used more responsibly because it costs to participate.

In a private system, the total dynamic is defined by the individual provider and the individual consumer themselves, one on one. The level of service, the amount of service and the fees are all decisions relegated to the patient provider interface. There would be no national forums, no Romanow Reports, no need for consultation with the collective for the system.

In our public system, the standards are largely uniform and universal, decided on a scale or a continuum, somewhere between societal demand and the collective's ability to pay. These spending decisions are made at cabinet tables. Cabinet tables decide on funding and write cheques. Service and allocation of funds to different health disciplines for the most part are decided by people in the actual health system, the providers.

The theme of discussion in this book is the concept of prorated patient participation in one's illness care and self-wellness initiatives. I will expound as I go through the text. **Patients should actively participate in the costs of their individual care. The one hundred and twenty-five billion dollar question is: how could this happen?**

Many of my comments relating to health care providers in the system may not be understood or appreciated by some; however, the Canadian Health Care System was intended for the people of Canada and not for any other group of people, either public, professional, private or political. *And the system is most definitely worth saving.*

CHAPTER 1

The Canadian Health Care System

We Canadians are blessed with an advanced society. We have peace, order, and good governance existing throughout a small social democracy with thirty-three million people in a vast land mass bounded by three oceans and two American borders, the Alaskan and the forty-ninth parallel states.

In 2002, Canada was rated the third most desirable country in the world in which to live. This was the second year in a row at third position having been in the first position in the world for the previous seven years. Colloquially speaking, "not too shabby" considering some one hundred and fifty countries were assessed by the United Nations for the annual index. In 2003, we have slipped to eighth place, still very respectable.

Throughout recent history, our great neighbor to the south has been a trusted guardian of our flank. We Canadians tend to compare ourselves to Americans with impunity and with a considerable lack of appreciation for our inherent differences. **We do this frequently in health.**

Many Canadians think the American system is superior to ours.

The recent rhetoric and nasty comments, popular and political, between Canadians and Americans is a testament to the continued and mounting difficulties between the two countries.

We two friendly neighbors, the only ones excluding Mexico and the French islands, in the North American land mass are viewed, ironically, in very different ways around the world. Canadians, of course, are viewed as the great peacemakers and keepers. We have a huge garnering of respect and trust universally, probably the highest in the world. Our southern neighbor, on the other hand, is for the most part viewed as the modern day economic imperialist and colonialist.

Unfortunately, despite a large amount of humanitarian activity around the globe, the Americans are viewed as interlopers, bullying and sometimes warmongering. The Americans apparently see themselves as "globo-cops" and self-appointed vigilantes of world peace. The current presidential acrimony does not seem to be helping anything: "If you are not with us you are against us!" **This is not the Canadian way.**

The distribution and redistribution of wealth in Canada is clearly more equitable than in the USA and is very similar to Norway and Sweden. These two Scandinavian countries were this year's first and second place finishers respectively in the U.N. index. Therein lies the substance of the attractive socio-economic situation in

Canada. **We are a benevolent social democracy with marvelous programs that make us a very socially advanced nation.** The interests and well being of the Canadian collective are fairly well balanced with the interests and well being of the individual. **Clearly our societal structure is one of the most outstanding in the world, and possibly in all of history.**

Our social programs have been developed by, if not demanded by, the people of Canada over the last 137 years since 1867. They are our greatest assets as a people since gaining our stripes with the proud tragedy at Vimy Ridge, France, as a forty-year-old country in the First Great War.

Canada: A Social Democracy

Canada is a progressive social democracy with egalitarianism born out of a broad breadth of population of middle class.

We have few very rich or very poor people on the continuingly narrowing left and right socio-economic tails of the bell curve.

Peaceful and just societies are spawned by redistribution of a land's wealth and Canada has done a masterful job at fine-tuning the elements of our society that protect all and everyone.

Canada guarantees a fair opportunity for a good quality of life to all people in the Canadian mosaic.

We have a quality, comprehensive Charter of Human Rights and Freedoms.

The Charter is solid and protects the individual from the collective and the converse, the collective from the individual.

Our executive, legislative and judicial branches can be changed with and by the will of the people regularly and as often as wanted and needed.

The social programs I refer to were born out of a demanding, critical, discerning, and righteous Canadian people.

Equal access to education, health, sustenance, housing and justice is guaranteed.

Freedom of movement, religion, press and speech, often taken for granted, is also guaranteed.

Freedom from harassment, incarceration, persecution and discrimination is guaranteed.

Labour laws and a universal no-fault insurance for our employers and employees are in place.

Employment insurance is available to bridge gaps in earnings.

All these are jewels of Canadian society and are for the most part taken for granted by many of our people.

Canadians have never known a different system, and many seem to think all the rest of the world is like today's Canada. It is of course not true. A very great majority of the world's population can only dream of living as well and as securely as Canadians in the most unfavourable situations. Just recently there was a decision by the State of Oregon to reject publicly funded health care. This was a cardinal manifestation of the difference between Canada and the United States. The health professionals of Oregon, doctors primarily, lobbied hard to prevent public health care.

The very critical and solicitous popular mindset these days of the Canadian people may now be the worst threat to our social programs, programs that we demanded as the great social equalizers of our advanced society.

Now Canadians are too critical of their health system. A large amount of the criticism of our social programs and the administration thereof is destructive, unfounded and exaggerated, endangering the very foundations of all our Canadian social systems.

We have one of the most just societies on earth.

The recent Program for International Student Assessment (PISA), done out of Paris for the Organization of Economic Cooperation and Development (OECD) countries showed Canada well above the ninetieth percentile compared to a large number of developed countries.

If Alberta and Ontario were countries, they would have the best education systems in the world based solely on student performance. Recently, Statistics Canada affirmed that we have the highest percentage of population **by far** blessed with post-secondary training **in the entire world.**

Canada's Health Care System: The Delivery

Our Health Care System is quite arguably, and is in my opinion, the best in the world.

Yet it is the brunt of much derisive criticism and uninformed comparison with **usually** the American system.

Unfortunately, the unrelenting criticism is coming mostly from service providers in the system, opposition politics, and opinions based on anecdotal episodes.

Much of the mal-opinion is based on unrealistic expectations. Our illness-based health care system is not able to do wellness promotion and disease prevention before the disease arrives.

Our illness-based system is overwhelmed with unprecedented individual wants as opposed to needs.

The poor opinion of our system is often based on the failure to understand that a publicly funded, universal no fault, no individual cost, social health care system has a corollary. That corollary simply stated is:

In a social health care system, those who can wait do wait and those who cannot wait do not wait.

This is fortunately the current situation, with many thanks to all the service providers in the system today who move the sickest patients to the front of the line by the hour with great integrity and fairness.

Canadians now want a system where nobody ever waits for anything.

Opportunists, be they service providers or various advocates, politicians or the private sector are using this issue to support self-interest. Inevitably, people in American private health care systems must wait as well, and they do. Sometimes patients in foreign private systems, regardless of degree of illness, wait much longer than patients in Canada. For many patients in developed foreign countries the wait time endured is not because some other patients are justifiably sicker, but because there are insufficient financial resources to buy faster service, or any service.

Secondly, foreign patients wait because there is far more bureaucratic entanglement in their health maintenance organizations, that often prevents and delays health care from being provided to the individual.

Oftentimes, enormous and impossible amounts of money have to be paid up front. This is before urgently needed health service will be provided for possible approval later by the insurance company. This is, for the most part, the unfortunate situation in the United States today.

Don't Trade It In: Fix It

The Canadian Health Care System has all the desirable features and very few of the undesirable features of a quality and a fair health care system.

The system was designed for the collective, but it is assessed by individual episodes and demands.

It is the best of all possible systems but with imperfections that the consumers and providers have criticized until the system is ready to collapse.

Clearly, a flat tire does not make an expensive car a lemon that needs to be traded in for a new, good model.

Like the tire on the car, our health care system needs change and adjustment not a new system or a parallel system.

All illness and frailty in society cannot be allayed, prevented, and treated immediately with the most desirable outcomes. This is an objective that cannot be attained with any amount of money. It is elementary that humans grow old and die and humans get sick and die. Our health care system can never be good enough to keep everyone in perfect health until the day they die! Society could not fund it collectively, and very few individuals in our society could fund it individually.

Wellness

It is clear that an individual who becomes very ill needs the help of the health care system to sort out or cure that illness.

It is also equally clear that the wellness and fitness of an individual in our country must be the responsibility of that individual, though fostered by social mores.

How could it be otherwise?

Individual wellness and fitness cannot be obtained through the health care system. But good fitness and wellness, individually attained, clearly will reduce the use of and therefore the financial strain on the Canadian Health Care System.

Which family or individual today is able to spend forty to fifty percent of all annual income on their health, even if not sick, as the provinces and territories do currently?

With the current growth rates, some provinces including our biggest, Ontario, are moving very rapidly, in the next two or three decades, to sixty or sixty-five percent.

Popular and professional opinion is that we should do this collectively when we could never do this individually.

The national and provincial presidents of large health professional organizations openly say "The system needs more money!" "It is under-resourced!"

One must remember that this amount of provincial-territorial government spending goes to illness, perceived illness and generated malady born out of poor lifestyle, and also sometimes for illicit monetary gain. Many people use the free health care system intensively and repetitively to obtain insurance pay-outs, government social support benefits and to pay off insured loans on everything one could imagine from homes to cars and boats.

A minuscule portion of the illness-based health care dollar goes to wellness.

Population wellness should not be attempted by spending in the illness-based health care system. This could be likened to taking a farm tractor to a formula one car race. Wrong vehicle, and wrong driver!

For instance, for whatever inconceivable reason, the Federal Department of Health is in charge of fitness! Fitness and wellness, for obvious reasons, have been almost totally forgotten by the Federal Department of Health.

Fitness and amateur sport should stand alone again as a Federal department and be adequately funded, possibly by money taken from health.

No amount of spending after the fact on diagnosed illness will have any effect on prevention of

illness. Only money spent on wellness will achieve the goal of wellness promotion and therefore illness prevention.

High blood pressure, diabetes and obesity have overwhelmed western society and will soon do the same in the developing world. The two primary and initial treatments for these mega health problems are exercise and appropriate diet. Doctors and pills come later. **Exercise and diet are education issues, not health issues.**

The health care system is not set up to teach prevention of illness and promotion of wellness.
First of all, it only sees sick people and those who think they are sick, excepting possibly in programs for pre and post-natal screening.

Secondly, wellness is an educational issue and should occur in the education systems where it can be delivered across the full spectrum to all people. It should be delivered at the right age and before fixed habits are set and when students are at the most impressionable age.

Wellness is not the absence of illness. If someone is not sick it does not mean they are well. Curing illness does not conceptually produce any population or individual wellness.

Health education and physical education adequately provided and valued intrinsically in our schools would do enormously more for population wellness than our health care system. A modern calculated and compulsory health education and physical education curriculum in our schools would most assuredly eventually curb costs in the health care system and increase productivity in society.

So why do we not do this?

Good question. **We westerners spend too much of our time generating our wealth instead of paying attention to our health and wellness.**

Despite **one hundred and twenty-five billion dollars a year** in global spending in the Canadian Health Care System,

despite nearly fifty percent of all annual provincial budgets,

despite health care costing ten percent of the Canadian Gross Domestic Product (G.D.P.),

our Canadian population wellness demographics are worse today in 2004 than they were ten years ago, and were worse then than ten years before that!

As stated above, the health care system, in spite of all this spending, does not produce much, if any, population wellness. It provides only relief and monitoring of illness with probably far too much zero and low-outcome results after medical intervention.

Indeed our public health system already does far more for population wellness and prevention of disease than the illness-based health care system could ever achieve.

Public health care initiatives such as immunization,

clean water, clean food and proper waste disposal have a much larger impact on population wellness than our illness-based health care system. Public safety issues, like salting and sanding roads and walkways, seat belts, bicycle helmets, radar detectors, breathalyzers and twinned highways have saved many lives and reduced emergency room trauma by a great margin. Orthopedics, for instance, once all about car accidents, trauma, and fractures is today far more about joint replacement procedures for degenerative disease. This is a result of public health and safety initiatives.

But Canada's population demographics on wellness today are ominous and worsening.

Obesity and inactivity will surely lead to more cardiovascular disease, many more cancers and increasing incidence of diabetes with all the ensuing complications.

These are complications of our advanced society and generate little public outcry for a problem that has far more implications for the health, wellness and productivity of Canadians than any inadequacy in the Canadian illness care system.

We should be applying further financial resources to health instruction and physical education in our schools and to activities in our communities rather than to the health care system.

More resource attention on the childhood years is needed in better balance with the resource attention being paid to the senior years.

It has been said that seventy percent of health care costs are consumed by the eldest thirty percent of the population. Possibly our social spending is imbalanced on an age parameter. Possibly too much is spent on the aged and not enough on our youth. This element of Canadian social policy should be reconsidered, even more especially when one sees so much pressure for deficit financing of health spending. In other words, health care today, paid for tomorrow by someone else, is basically socially wrong.

Interest on the federal debt annually is about thirty-five billion, about half of the annual health care spending by all governments. Essentially, deficit spending in health translates to our grandchildren paying years later for our blood pressure checks and our medications that we receive today. As Wimpy says in the Popeye cartoons: "I will gladly pay you tomorrow for a hamburger today." I don't think so, Tim.

Where Will the Money Come From?

In the following chapters, I would like to give my impression of where we were in health care, where we are now, and where we should be going in the future.

There is not much 'horse-sense' in health dollars.

Health dollars are consumed oftentimes with impunity, with greed, with ignominy, with the self-righteousness of the taxpayer, with little or no relation to outcomes, and with little or no regard for any cost benefit analysis.

In effect we have achieved optimum and excellent health care for those truly ill patients in the system, who really need treatment, by giving broad attentive over-care to all and anyone in society who wants it but may not need it. We do not need to burn down the pig barn to get a roast of pork!

The health care system is craving and demanding more service and therefore more money, very obviously.

Where is this money to come from? Ultimately, there are only three possible sources: The collective tax base, the individual consumer, or both.

So again, where should the *extra* money come from? What social formula should be used for its extraction from the Canadian population or possibly from the consumer individually? I will address this later in the text.

If we do not make the correct decisions in this next short while, then the Canadian health system will most definitely move into full duality – one public system and one private.

Tiering or multiple levels of care in both systems will also occur. We will have not only two tiers, but multi-tiers in both systems.

This would be, and surely will be, a colossal shame. Many developed social democratic countries that have gone this route, freely admit today that the change to duality was not for the better.

These countries, such as Sweden, the United Kingdom, New Zealand, Ireland and more, have moved to the dual multi-tiered systems because their tax bases could not sustain the uncontrolled utilization and growth in public spending. **They hit the 'fiscal wall' and many of Canada's provinces will soon do so with certainty.** Their public systems in effect became the less desirable systems of last resort with overflow into the private system if one could afford to pay.

Note: The Romanow Report is only eighteen months old as I write and seems forgotten. The Premier of British Columbia wants another meeting, for a week, with the other Premiers to plan the reform of health care!

As stated earlier, projections indicate that the current growth rates in health spending, in twenty years or so will see some provinces spending sixty or more percent of all annual budgets on health. **This cannot and will not happen.** This would leave only forty percent or less for all other government programs.

Of course, this presumes status quo and does not include any expansions of Medicare.

Note: Mr. Romanow is currently suggesting that we should fund programs beyond hospital care and physician costs, to include program proposals for long-term care and pharmacare. **Where will the money come from?**
Our problem in Canadian health care is most definitely not a marginal lack of funding, but massive over-utilization.

Many medical services in the Canadian Health Care System are not needed and not indicated. The system is being used when it should not be used. This is over-utilization. It is a large cost factor and a large waste of financial resources.

Utilization may best be described as the amount of usage the health system gets.

How much health care utilization, or services rendered or given to patients, should not occur, is not needed, or could be done by alternate less expensive providers? A large amount in my estimation.

The argument about which level of government should cover what percentage of costs is an issue, but **our health care system can conceivably and easily consume all provincial budgets in their entirety over time.** *So why are we not addressing utilization?* Culling out the nonsense health care makes eminent sense. Is it because patients are voters to politicians, and financial gold mines to service providers of every sort?

Defining the Problem

I feel strongly that we have not defined the basic problem with the system.

Health spending of this magnitude without monitoring utilization and outcomes does not pass the sanity test. Therefore, all solutions conjured up and applied to date have failed. Mr. Romanow's solution will have the same fate.

I am reminded of the story of two guys who started a business. They purchased a truck and were buying potatoes for fifty cents a pound in one region and hauling them to another region to be sold for one dollar a pound. Their cost of transportation and operation was fifty cents a pound. After six months things were not very good as you can imagine.

One guy said to the other: "We need to do something."

He agreed and said: "Yes, we need to buy a bigger truck."

If we do not define the problem, chances are we will not find the solution.

The providers in the system, the health care professionals of every sort, continue to berate the system with considerable acerbic public volume and presence. The refrain is continuous: **The health system is in crisis and collapsing; add more money, sixty-five percent of which, of course, is salaries.**

Fortunately, inside the much over-utilized health care system is a condensed system, a core system addressing the needs of the truly ill and injured as opposed to the "walking well". Largely, this core system is at higher levels of care or at the secondary and tertiary levels of care; care given, for the most part, by specialists.

This core system is as good quality as the best health care delivery in the world, *for the Canadians who are truly ill and injured.*

Unfortunately, its quality is clouded, disguised, masked and overwhelmed by significant over-utilization, missutilization, marginal abuse, and incessant calculated provider criticism delivered with great credibility to the population.

This core system is now starting to unravel.

The providers in the system do an excellent and superlative job of triaging or selecting out the truly ill and injured for more rapid and intensive delivery of care.

In this manner, therefore, they protect the core system, so to speak.

Over-utilization of health care, however, I judge to be driven seventy-five percent by the consumers and twenty-five percent by the providers.

Over-utilization may represent as much as twenty-five percent of all service volume and is, in my estimation, the main problem. Throughout the system, nearly all of this over-utilization is for the most part inadvertent and now socially customary and acceptable. **It is free right! Therefore it has no relative value.**

Sustainability is a cardinal and key health-care catchword today. There are fourteen governments with fourteen departments of health and fourteen departments of finance that are plagued and challenged on a daily basis by this word, sustainability. **Are we able to afford our health care system?**

These fourteen all have tried to balance the financial realities of governments and the volatility in health with the daily political realities. Patients are voters and voters are patients as stated above. There has been much complaining about the system, public and professional, political and partisan. Blame for the difficulties in health care has been fired in all directions with increasing federal-provincial conflict, inter-provincial acrimony and provider-government arguing.

Caught up in the middle, the people of Canada have stated clearly: Enough already! Just fix it and stop the ballyhoo!

Fixing it will mean both decreasing utilization and sorting out the shared funding arrangements and principles, both for governments and consumers.

Sustainability, Affordability, Utilization, Accountability

To be able to keep our public health care system and make it sustainable, we must make it affordable.

We must be able to pay for it without affecting all other government programs, such as transportation, economic development, education, tourism and others.

To be able to afford the public health care system, we must all work together to make it efficient, and it must be used properly by all. Obviously **this means utilization controls.**

> **Sustainability is all about affordability.**
> **Affordability is all about utilization.**
> **Utilization is all about patient and provider accountability.**
> **Accountability of the patient is all about 'patient participation' in costs.**

In other words, are our governments able to continue to pay, through tax collected, for our health care costs? Affordability directly determines sustainability.

Accountability refers to the responsibility that patients and providers have to use the system correctly and only when needed.

How do we instill accountability in patients and providers?

The definition of the problem appears to me to be more about the patient's financial participation in utilization than anything else. The large, political, public, acrimonious debate between the federal government and its provinces and territories is irrelevant.

What does patient participation mean? I will start by saying what it does not mean.

It does not mean user fees!

It does not mean duality!

It does not mean denial of service to the poor.

It does not mean that a patient needs money to be seen by a provider.

Originally, Medicare was designed to prevent catastrophic costs to a patient and allow free and equal access to physicians' services and hospital care. In the early eighties the Canada Health Act eliminated any extra billing by Canadian physicians. Indeed at the time, the federal government promoted the Canada Health Act politically by saying to the public, "Patients will never receive another doctor's bill." They stashed the announcement nicely, I remember, in the "baby bonus" or Family Allowance cheque envelope.

Now we have the odd situation of the Canada Health Act precluding private health care in that some patients now want to buy faster health care service in Canada and buying it is illegal because selling it is illegal. Some people go to the United States of America to purchase faster **but not better** health care for a variety of reasons. In Canada, health care insured under Medicare is not allowed to be sold; therefore, then, it cannot be purchased.

So then how do we address the over-utilization issue in Canadian health care and continue to prevent catastrophic costs for the individual and ensure no financial barrier to entry or access to the health care system? *How do we take the health care system off life support?*

Medicare is an insurance, an insurance governed by federal legislation, the Canada Health Act. However, it is operated with full jurisdiction by the provinces and territories, a somewhat, if not completely, unworkable arrangement. A non-system of fourteen jurisdictions. Medicare ignores and defies all the basic principles of insurance and also the basic principles of human behavior.

The basic universal principle of insurance is one of client participation, or a deductible amount to be borne by the client: a deterrent. Human behavior encourages overuse and over consumption if "it is cost free". **The public concept that all health care is free and may be used at will must change.** If food was free, people would eat more. If car washing was free, there would be more car washing. **Health care is free and it is categorically overused.**

Note: There is paltry if any pertinent data collection in the Canadian Health Care System. Amazingly, we cannot afford to collect data adequately. What data we do have, we do not use well. Therefore we have virtually no solid actuarial figures to define or account for expenditures or utilization. The system is totally open-ended, come one, come all, and is based on the ill-defined principles of the Canada Health Act.

Canadians have an insatiable and infinite demand for publicly funded health care.

Many professional providers criticize the system but quietly enjoy its monetary benefits while espousing the quality of their individual care and the lack of quality of care provided by the system! Of course, when any individual patient's care is delayed or goes awry, it is never caused by virtue of patient over-utilization or rushed delivery of service. It is the fault of government under-funding that is the root cause, despite spending that is approaching fifty percent of every province's total budget!

Logically then, the Canada Health Act needs to be redefined. But redefined based on what values and principles? Surely not those values and principles that exist today, or the unfettered wants of each and every individual.

Clearly we want to have everything for everybody at all times in the health care system. Furthermore, we want it all as decided by the consumer, with no responsibility on the consumer.

Equally, there is no responsibility for utilization control and no incentive to deter or decrease utilization that can be delivered through the professionals who provide health services.

The general insurance industry today, in effect, demands or inflicts consumer behavior and responsibility by having consumer financial participation in the process. But even this industry is under duress because of mounting health claims for personal injury. **Repairing the car has become cost irrelevant!**

Where Do We Go From Here?

I believe that the current Canadian Health Care System can be sustained and maintained as a public system with prorated patient participation. Simple personal individual accountability.

What we need to do now in Canada is to redefine the Canada Health Act, by defining what is medically necessary, and defining patient participation; patient participation that ensures and guarantees two important basic provisions. Number one is the preservation of **barrier free access.** No money would be seen anywhere or be needed to get access to the system. **Number two is the universal protection from catastrophic costs.**

This concept of prorated patient participation **would address utilization in a meaningful way.** People would be more motivated to take ownership of their health and the health of their loved ones to save cost. **This concept would also greatly stimulate and motivate patient participation in self-wellness, health promotion and disease prevention.** Fewer people would irrationally continue to dig their graves with their teeth! Self-wellness initiatives would be inherent in the process and would further evolve with time.

I believe that patients should participate in the cost of all their health care. This participation would be prorated or adjusted to income. No cash would ever be seen or used in the system. High-income earners would pay more and low-income earners would pay less; some would pay nothing at all. All would have a maximum annual contribution beyond which the public system would pay all.

I believe, based on experience, that this concept of patient participation in their costs of consumption of health care could reduce overall use of the

health care system and reduce resulting costs by a minimum of fifteen percent.

Fifteen percent of the portion of health spending that is public expenditure, which is in the vicinity of ninety billion dollars, represents very nearly fifteen billion dollars annually in reduced costs. Worth a think tank at least, I believe.

Note: Mr. Romanow and Mr. Kirby amazingly did not even talk about the demand side of health care, only the supply side. Open the tap wider! As if everything going on in the health care system now is justified, absolutely necessary, and furthermore we need more of it and it will make a difference!

CHAPTER 2

The Business of Health Care

In Canada today, our publicly funded health care has numerous unappreciated benefits and values. They have been taken for granted by many Canadians.

Many benefits, unseen and unappreciated, are taken for granted as if they were and will always be there. If one were to ask a Swedish person or a New Zealander if it were possible for a fully publicly-funded open-ended health system like Canada's to collapse, they would say, "You bet it can!" Theirs did! It can happen readily here in Canada as well, either rapidly or piecemeal by province. Any sustained economic downturn plus high interest rates would make several of our provinces very unstable financially.

Health care in Canada is a one hundred and twenty-five billion dollar a year industry with plenty of profit.

In Canada, the private spending accounts for about

thirty percent, the public spending is the rest, or seventy percent. **Private spending is spending by individuals that does not fall under Medicare paid by governments,** for example, optometry, physiotherapy, and some medication. **Public spending is the expenditures made by all governments under Medicare.** *There is profit on virtually all spending.*

The private spending, forty billion or thereabouts, is for the most part covered by some sort of private insurance. In many cases, it is covered through the work place of the patient.

The business and mercantile sector in Canada enjoys considerable benefit from the publicly-funded Canadian Health Care System. It takes care of the health of their Canadian employees at no direct cost to the business sector, a significant advantage over the Americans.

The cost of employee health to the employers of Canada in a postulated pure private health care system would be difficult to estimate. Surely, though, it would be more than significant and similar to the huge costs in the United States.

In the United States, fifteen percent or more of the people do not have any sort of health care coverage, very nearly fifty million people in the "land of the free and the home of the brave." Many more have inadequate coverage. Their places of employment do not provide such insurance and the cost of individual coverage is far too expensive.

These fifty million Americans, when ill, now have to rely on charity or divestiture of some or all things owned in order to pay their health care bill. Sometimes their relatives even have to divest pensions, mortgage homes or borrow. Some people go back to work having already been retired, in order to pay for illness or injury in the family.

Roy Romanow recently said, "For the political people to say, we're not buying it, we haven't got the money, or we can't do that, I think that is a prescription for political suicide." What about financial suicide? It seems to me that financial suicide is more significant than political suicide.

A Political Response

Politics, business and health care are obviously intertwined. With respect, in essence, Mr. Romanow has avoided a very major issue. He has recommended only more spending without also addressing the cardinal problem of over-utilization. Again, we are attempting to solve the problem by writing a cheque. That is not too profound. Wrong diagnosis! Wrong treatment! **When you ask a politician to do a job then you will undoubtedly get a political result or answer.**

When the only tool one has is a hammer, everything looks like a nail!

We need a non-political answer to the health care challenges in Canada *now*, or we will lose the system.

The Canadian voter, if not informed properly, will not support a government that suggests rationalization of their health care system. To the voter, more money means better health care and the providers of course will always agree.

The money removed from health by the federal government in the middle nineties needs to go back into the system, without any doubt, if people's health care expectations remain the same. However, utilization controls will have been again totally ignored.

The two billion dollars just recently added to the health care system by the federal government has been described as "a drop in the bucket". Big bucket! We need to avoid kicking the health care bucket.

The people of Canada need to know that more money put into the health system may lead to its collapse.

I had the experience a few years ago of seeing a five year-old child with a sore throat and a fever early one morning. I sent the child to our rural hospital for some investigation because of some soft and subtle signs. He was too sick for a sore throat.

After noon I had a call from the laboratory. A diagnosis of acute leukemia was made by the lab technician. Moments later I spoke to the parents. They had only two questions. Number one, "Where can we get the best?" Number two, "How soon can we get it?"

The answers to these two questions in Canada are easy for every doctor and every set of parents. The answer to number one is, "Right around here!" and to question number two "Later today or tomorrow morning!"

Indeed the best pediatric care in the world is available from Victoria to St. John's and in many, many places in between. How long will it take to get the care? As long as it takes to drive or fly there; that is how soon here in Canada.

With time, the child did well and has had the usual tough period of chemotherapy resulting in a remission that has to date led to an anxious cure.

A similar situation in the private health system in the United States of America would not generate only these two questions. There would be more. Mom and Dad would certainly have a third and a fourth. "Where will we find the money? Will our insurance cover all the costs?"

Conceivably, the costs could be two, three or four hundred thousand dollars (US) to take care of their child. Not finding the resources would result in a profound guilt trip for the family unparalleled in a lifetime. For many families, the care of their loved one who is sick or injured leaves the family financially devastated. *A full thirty percent of the personal bankruptcies in the USA on an annual basis occur as a result of someone in the family getting sick or having an accident.*

As stated above, the Americans spend fifty percent more on health care per capita as a percent of gross domestic product than Canadians. **Is applying more money to the Canadian Health Care System the answer? A cautious "yes" at this particular point in time, in that the Canadian Health Care System is somewhat under-funded in selective areas for what it is being currently asked to do. But there has to be more than just more money.**

Recently, a couple I know traveled to the southern USA to "buy some sun". During the vacation, the male had an episode of unstable angina and obviously a heart attack was impending. He went to a hospital and had a rather rapid quadruple coronary by-pass. In the recovery room, he had a blood leak or bleed of one of the by-pass grafts. He was rushed back to the operating room for another operation for immediate repair.

Subsequently, in the cardiac intensive care unit, he had an acute onset of kidney failure as a result of the episode or period of rather long critical illness. He was in a Cardiac Care Unit for twenty-one days before being discharged and being able to return home to Canada.

Price tag? Two hundred and sixty thousand dollars, US!

Between the two surgeries and during the first twenty-four hours, the spouse was "obligated" to immediately find a ten thousand dollar US deposit! Try to make those actuarial figures fit any insurance program. Which rich person would want these costs in a private health care system with premiums to pay accordingly? This kind of insurance is virtually impossible with the large and increasing incidence of heart disease.

This kind of thing is unheard of in Canada, *but only unheard of as yet!* Listen a little bit longer! *It may well happen.*

Which system would you choose?

Does the Canadian system deserve the relentless destructive criticism it is receiving? I think not.

Again, a large portion of the criticism is coming from our providers. Almost always, the criticism is delivered to the public via the press. Physicians' ongoing criticism of the Medicare system is frequently given directly to patients and is also a large pervading negative factor. Criticism also comes from hospital board members, administrators, nurses, allied health professionals, unionized health care workers and politically motivated people. All have personal agendas that are rolled out under the guise and complaint of an existing poor health care system and the need for more money and therefore improvement of health care. Correct? No.

The Canadian Medical Association continues to suggest that more resources need to be added to the health system and requests to be present "at the table", to defend the Canadian people. It is ludicrous to suggest that the Canadian people need to be defended or protected from their elected governments. In a democracy, the people can defend themselves against governments but not against special interest groups. The people can throw a government out at an election but cannot throw out a special interest group at any time.

If forty-five percent of all provincial spending going on health is not enough, then what is enough?

Why does the Canadian Medical Association not suggest to its members, and to consumers, rationalization maneuvers on the demand side? Cost effectiveness. Cost controls. Why do they not speak out against walk-in clinics? Why do they not speak out against questionable indications for many health services and procedures?

What table is it that they want to be at? Advocacy and advisory roles of Canadian physicians are now already very much alive and very effective. They obviously cannot be at the cabinet tables of Canada where the people's tax money is allocated.

The Canadian people cannot afford what the Canadian Medical Association seems to be advocating: more resources but no demand-side rationalization.

All health care providers have a resoundingly similar rhyme. "The government should be doing something!" "We need more of us and more money in the system." As well, the resulting *or else* alternative frequently quoted is inevitably, "People will surely die because of the government's ineptitude and for the lack of health resources." Crisis! The rhetoric goes on, magnified prior to each successive negotiation and election.

The solutions proposed inevitably are about "quantity". Increased quantity of dollars and increased quantity of providers will ensure quality of care. We usually do not hear that quality assurance principles and accountability procedures will determine the quantity of dollars that need to be spent and the numbers of human resources that are needed.

Just as one's bank account balance is more often than not about spending than earning, health care sustainability is now more about frivolous utilization than increased resources of any sort.

If a fellow passenger getting on an airliner informed another passenger that the plane and the airline were not adequate and therefore unsafe, that passenger would probably ignore the comment. If an airline employee at the gates, and if one of the pilots and the attendants all said the airline was not adequate and therefore unsafe, the passenger might well have a different assessment of the situation.

Governments are unable to deal rationally and effectively with these sorts of intense political pressures.

I reiterate: for many provinces and territories, soon the entire provincial-territorial budgets for health may exceed fifty percent of all spending. How can this not be enough? What will be enough? As well, spending continues to grow like a proverbial weed, sixty-five percent of the money going to people in the system as salary and benefits.

The Americans spend fifty percent more per capita on health care than Canadians.

A very large part of this money in the USA comes from the employers of the country. Although American corporate tax is twenty percent compared to Canada's at thirty percent, mostly private-for-profit insurance companies and health maintenance organizations of all sorts manage American health care, and the cost of doing business is high. Overhead is passed directly on to the patient/consumer and is paid through wage deductions. Inevitably, the cost of health insurance is many hundreds of dollars per month per individual.

Individuals with poor family medical histories or those who exhibit existing disease have difficulty getting employed. Pre-employment medical checks are often mandatory, stringent and exclusive, preventing employment. It has been said that a large automobile manufacturer in America spends more on health care for its employees than on steel for operations.

There is a categorical difference between a public health care system and a private health care system. Both systems in parallel I call duality, not two tiers. We have two tiers now based on our individual province's ability to pay per capita. Some provinces are able to spend significantly more per capita than others. Canadians will not accept one system for the rich and one system for others, a fact confirmed by the Romanow Report.

Unfortunately, **Canadians, including many health**

professionals, do not understand the difference be-tween a private health care system and a public sys-tem with private provision of care.

Indeed, most physicians in Canada right now are and historically were private. Physicians' practices are private business where the patients are insured publicly. The ambulance that is called is also very likely to be pri-vate. Pharmacy is private. Unfortunately and unneces-sarily, MRI is sometimes private. The federal government spoke out, prior to the last election, against private MRI clinics and amazingly supports private abortion clinics.

Then why all the "to do" about the Alberta private hospital initiative? It was only yesterday, figuratively, that there were hundreds of private hospitals in the Canadian system run by the religious orders and benevolent organi-zations. They were all private or part and part. I should think profit has six letters and not four. Surely in capitalist North America, profit cannot be portrayed as a bad thing. The most profitable business in North America I suspect may very well be health care. Physicians, nurses, all other health professionals, pharmacies, suppliers of technology, software, hardware and so on all generate profit. I do not know of any provider or corporate structure that provides a health service or a product for only cost, no profit.

The concept of private service in a public system is fine. It may help to augment and evolve the system's over-all capability to provide services. But again, agencies that operate for profit, I feel, will not do much to prevent the existing significant system stress of over-utilization. **Over-utilization, I repeat, is the crux of the problem in the**

Canadian Health Care System.

The private hospital concept that is now frequently promoted by some and oftentimes condemned by others, assumes that all funding, even with a profit margin, is coming from the tax base, which, therefore, means that this remains a public system; health care is therefore being privately provided, yet in a singular publicly-funded system. Interestingly, this concept does not contravene the Canada Health Act, but obviously will not be welcomed by public employees.

Comparing the Canadian and U.S. Models: Private vs. Public

Our Canadian model is not at all similar to the American model and should not be compared.

Frequently, I have been asked to describe the difference between the Canadian public, and American private, health systems. Sometimes I launch into a large involved description. Sometimes I say, *"In Canada we provide health care; in the United States they sell health care."* Clearly a different mind-set.

The price tag for health care in Canada is somewhat controlled with great difficulty by governments. The price tag for health care in the USA is basically all that the market will bear. That is fifty percent more than in Canada per capita, as mentioned above.

Some Canadian doctors and nurses cannot work in the American 'wallet biopsy' monetary milieu.

In 1989, the then American First Lady and many others in the United States promoted the Hilary Clinton Medicare Initiative. ***Mrs. Clinton stated that the American health system should be like that in Canada.*** That was the theme. Interestingly, I was interviewed on the issue by one of her workers.

Mrs. Clinton's initiative did not happen of course, largely because the American Medical Association and other providers derailed it as a result of an aggressive well-organized national lobby.

The Business of Medicine: Quality of Service

Currently, I feel that many of our Canadian doctors may be shifting more and more towards an American pure business mentality. The traditional ministry of medicine is shifting to the business of medicine. Missionary to mercenary, physician dedication and devotion now more than ever seems only to come for a price. The Canadian health-provider establishment frequently looks at their governments as the common enemy. Unfortunately, they do not even see our governments as the elected purveyors acting on behalf of the people, administering their most valued social program. **Everybody working in the system categorically claims to know better than government about everything except controlling costs!**

On the physician side of health human resources, there are no negotiated designated medical services that would have to, or should have to, stay in place during strikes. Strikes, work stoppages and slow-downs are not uncommon now, and full or partial withdrawal of medical services with no legislative rules, regulations, agreements or consequences to deal with them haunt our legislators. This soon has to be dealt with by all provincial governments. Governments effectively are totally emasculated in the face of these developments in the negotiation process.

The upsets a few years ago in the province of Quebec's emergency rooms and in Newfoundland and British Columbia are ideal examples of a non-functioning relationship between governments and the private medical professionals in the provision of health care. In these provinces, doctors withdrew services and confronted governments. **The medical profession has used its ultimate "weapon", and the governments of Canada will certainly use theirs as well: legislation.**

What are the alternatives? How can we put together a public delivery system with private provision of health care services within it, and make it work, when nothing is clearly defined on paper with physicians, and there are no legal arrangements? This is a critical factor and one of the most salient flaws in the Canadian Health Care System.

Doctors are almost all private-for-profit and independent of the system. Governments could solve this by making all doctors employees of government. No more private practice. This change would be volcanic, eruptive and disruptive. There would be many negative consequences, most predominantly in rural Canada. However, there is now some considerable passive movement in this direction, especially by younger physicians in large urban areas.

A balance might be struck if governments were to negotiate minimum service standards in the event of physician strikes. But negotiate with whom? Physicians do not answer to their professional organizations. The professional organizations negotiate pay on behalf of physicians but have absolutely no control over the physicians' individual or collective actions. If every physician in a province wanted or decided collectively to take the same week off, they could, and increasingly they would.

Professional medical organizations across Canada are now, in essence, acting like unions and are being viewed as such by governments. However, there are no ground rules. If the medical community is to act in effect like unions, that demand the societal privilege of striking, then society must have the protection of rules and regulations about this sort of "union" activity. Expect governments to legislate to solve their problems.

Years ago, the "old school" medical community often stated that the ultimate negotiation weapon or tool, withdrawal of service or strike, was too ominous and too heavy-handed to use. Today, withdrawal of medical service and the threat of it are quite common as stated above. Sometimes it is selective, sometimes for a day, sometimes for longer. Medical service strikes and the threat of strikes are occurring with increasing frequency in Canada. Settlements have been large as a result of one province's physicians threatening to go to another and the converse. **The facts are that few physicians move and very few go to the USA.** Equally, **very few patients go to the USA despite the vast amount of ink this marginal activity gets awarded in the press.**

Making the Patient Accountable

Then how do the people of Canada resolve this worsening impasse?

In the health care triangle: patient, provider and insurer, business principles are observed only very sparingly and only marginally on the side of the triangle that runs between doctor and government. What about the patient? Is it possible for the patient to effect a rational change throughout the whole triangle, given that the providers and insurers seem to have failed? I believe the answer to this question is yes.

Patients must be included in the business side of their health care. But how could this occur? And how should it occur?

Simply, the patient must be able to assess value given for the cost of service.

But the patient usually thinks the service provided for him or her is cost free and of no personal financial value!

The patient also thinks, when asked, that fees paid out on their behalf to their physician are many times the actual fee.

Patients also quietly accept expeditious service because there is an alleged shortage of doctors.

But the patient, he or she, is not involved! No authority! No import! No accountability!

The debate all across this country, post Romanow, about accountability should be about patient-doctor accountability, and not about government-to-government accountability. Governments are arguing incessantly about who is accountable. The federal government is chastising the provinces, stating publicly that they are misappropriating health dollars. **But there is no real accountability *now* between the doctor and the patient *and there should be.***

Is there a way to bring this irrationality to some rationality? I think the answer here is also yes. For instance, if a patient is dissatisfied with the quality or quantity of a service rendered by a physician, then the question arises, should it be automatically fully paid out with no question on the patient's behalf by the insurer (government)?

Today, no matter how quick or poor the quality of a service that is delivered by a physician, it is paid immediately in full, no questions asked. Try that in the restaurant business! That system is unparalleled in the business sector. The business sector should be so lucky as to have one hundred percent of accounts receivable regardless of quality. We reward the poor and irresponsible doctor and therefore punish the good and responsible ones.

The concept of patient empowerment would equalize, to a large degree, the balance of authority and power between physicians and patients. It is called accountability, a good thing.

I think that patients have very little power in the current system. They should be empowered. The principal is sound but it would need clearly defined guidelines.

As a basic principle, what would be wrong with empowering the consumer, the patient? It would definitely help in eliminating some of the utilization excesses on the physician's side of the service triangle.

Following suit, what maneuvers then are possible to institute on the patient side of the triangle, to help control patient over-utilization? Over-utilization is the critical problem and is chronically avoided in our recurring health system reviews. Roy Romanow gave it little or no attention; patients are also voters.

Patients do not, for the most part, like waiting or ex-"spending" time for health care. They do not want to expend any money, but they will "spend" time waiting grudgingly and quietly because they are not in a position to argue or complain. If and when they do complain about waiting, inevitably they are told "It is the government's fault" or, less frequently "Get another doctor". This is becoming all too commonplace.

Today, the trend for many family doctors and for specialists to a smaller degree, is to select with an interview their new patients. This is unacceptable. I know of a specialist doctor who started a timer when he began the consultation with a patient and stopped the interview when it rang! In the Code of Ethics of the Canadian Medical Association, this surely borders on the unethical.

The Canadian Medical Association's Code of Ethics states: Do not discriminate against any patient on such grounds as age, gender, marital status, medical condition, national or ethnic origin, physical or mental disability, political affiliation, race, religion, sexual orientation, or socioeconomic status. This does not abrogate the physician's right to refuse to accept a patient for legitimate reasons.

What factors, then, are assessed in these so-called practice entrance interviews? Is it the amount of illness? Is it the amount of submissiveness to the provider, the age of the patient, or maybe the patient's personality? Is it the amount of projected care needed per visit by the patient? Who was that guy Hippocrates, again? Now astoundingly, we are hearing, not frequently but occasionally, that if a patient has not been in to see his or her physician for a year or two, they may be taken off the practice list! **Punishing patients for being well is completely unacceptable.**

Volumization

In principle the reply often given to patients by providers that "It is the government's fault" may also be somewhat correct. **Governments are also at fault.** The large volume of medical services is a large quiet culprit. **Governments are quietly happy with everyone working at maximum capacity and volume.** The large volume of medical services is currently our only utilization control and is described often as a soft control of costs or a soft cap. In principle, then, if maximum volumization is our only decent method to control costs, the so-called hourglass phenomenon, then wait lists are clearly useful. Wait lists for physicians' services, bed occupancy, and access to machine technology, for instance, are inherent to the systems' function and as stated above are a soft cap on services. **There is,** of course, **no wait list for emergency service in Canada,** *yet.*

On the physician side, **the fee for service system clearly does drive volume and therefore costs.** There is no doubt that this is a large component of some physicians' practices. Those who operate their primary care practices for rapid-flow volume, simplicity and facility of patient care, abuse the system. Frequently, they average five minutes a patient visit.

Physicians have three routes for patients to take.
The first option is diagnosis and prescription; the second option is to review and refer to secondary care; and the third is to review and investigate.

Oftentimes, only one complaint is allowed per visit! "The right shoulder only today. You will have to make another appointment for the left one."

Not all physicians in primary care operate in this

fashion, but the number who do is major and is on the increase. Low office-visit fees historically have pushed volumization. Also, patients all too frequently want to have immediate specialist's care instead of primary care. This is also pushing volumization.

Complaints of a generalized shortage of primary care physicians also allows some doctors considerable complicity in moving unacceptable volumes of patients through. For some reason, the size of general practices may vary from seven or eight hundred patients, with frequent rotation, to five thousand or more patients and less frequent rotation. Some practices see their patients two times per year on average, some as high as five times per year on average.

Walk-in clinics create massive cross-practice duplication of patient loads. Dozens of family doctors in a single location, and maybe more, share patients with walk-in clinics: the family doctor for the fast "stuff", and the walk-in clinic doctor for faster "stuff". And it pays the same! Of course this is probably patient acceptable when the patient is not paying and is not truly sick.

Some patients who attend walk-in clinics for a full fee are actually told to go to their family doctor if they need a blood test or anything even slightly serious or complicated, or if they need follow-up; in other words, if they are sick. A full fee is paid for no service, no obligation.

Patients are often triaged or sent back out the door by reception staff if they are visibly ill or have

serious complaints specified as not for walk-in clinics. Nurses, of course, cannot do this in emergency rooms!

The price tag is the same for such unacceptable care as for a thorough general-practice visit. The physicians who do good comprehensive primary care are indirectly financially punished. Physicians who do high-rotation, pre-primary care, or Mac-medicine, are rewarded. Volumization is firmly justified by some physicians with defensive posturing. "Shortages are caused by government ineptitude," they say. Thus, the situation of delivering expeditious and poor service to patients for the same price as delivering good care and service continues to be rationalized.

This situation allows some physicians to consolidate and condense earnings into a shorter workweek and workday. Medical needs of patients outside these business hours are the government's responsibility in the minds of these providers. Their patients usually end up after hours the responsibility of an emergency room physician colleague. In some small cities and towns, twenty or thirty practices may have to be covered at night, Saturday and Sunday by a single emergency room physician. No wonder the emergency rooms are plugged!

Many primary care physicians, however, do have group on-call schedules to cover after hours. A large majority do not bother. Resultant angry patients, who wait long hours at emergency rooms for their medically urgent but simple needs versus medically emergent needs, are inevitably told it is the fault of Medicare, "It's government."

Quality of physician life is also cited as a reason for non-coverage of their practice after hours. Dozens of trades, professions and other jobs would not dare use this defense and yet they still work as many hours as many urban and some rural general practitioners. In the reality of a competitive market world, these other jobs would fail if one attempted to work only business hours. "Go to my competitor after hours when I am not available!"

Again, how do we make the Medicare system fit the real actual patient and public needs rather than the needs and wants of the professionals?

Patient focus. Not provider focus, in other words.

The business model can be the only option. Patient participation in the triangular process.

The medical profession soundly and consistently complains about losing physician independence: "Government is interfering in the doctor-patient relationship." Government clearly needs to interfere *now,* not in the medical side but in the business or value-for-services-provided side.

"Quality and proper health care will be compromised because of government interference" is often the physician's refrain. The simple facts are that since "government – the people" got involved in health care forty years ago, care is light years better than previously for the global population, the patient and the doctor as well.

Volumization has suited that element of the medical profession that would use it to earn large incomes, give poor and rapid service and give the public the impression and excuse that there is no choice. "Medicare is a poor system that government, the politicians, put in place. We have no choice but to move fast."

I believe that our Medicare is still a good system being much misused, because it is devoid of basic principles that address the frailty of human behavior. **We should fix it by eliminating useless utilization. We should fix it and not nix it for the incredible and frequently voiced "lack of money" defense.**

The volumization phenomenon is the product of all three sides of the triangle. The physician is not squeaky clean. Neither is the government. Nor are the patients squeaky clean either.

All three sides are complicit and benefit from this situation. The system has only one solution that fits all, correct? You guessed it! Government needs to continue to add more money, write a bigger cheque! That will surely fix it! Right? Wrong!

Patients drive volume significantly. They are the biggest drivers of volumization and their participation is significant and expensive. Many services deemed medically of no value by professionals are quite valuable in the eyes of the patient. For instance, annual check-ups, prostate specific antigen screening, low back x-rays, monthly cholesterol checks, obstetrical ultra-sounds for gender, and brain scans for classical migraine.

A big issue today is soft-tissue neck pain after automobile accidents. Pain persists and visits to the doctor continue incessantly until the "green poultice" is put on, oftentimes clearing up the pain instantly. The automobile insurance industry continues to struggle with this issue.

Patients try to build a "case" for Canada Pension, a "case" for Workers' Compensation, a "case" because of an inattentive spouse. Patients visit the doctor for letters for school absence after the fact, letters for work absence after the fact, and of course the "biggie" prescription refills on a monthly, bi-monthly or tri-monthly basis. These are only a few of the many useless, ulterior and non-illness related reasons that patients visit their doctors.

Also, **public advocacy drives utilization.** Television, women's magazines, men's magazines, newspapers, educational media, and a horde of other media promote utilization. "Everyone should get their male pap test." "Everyone should get a mammogram." "Get your cholesterol checked." And others too numerous to mention – Be health care solicitous and live long. **Longevity comes from the health care system. Correct? No!**

The Vision of Medicare

The Medicare system was set up to react to the onset of illness as it was defined in pre-Medicare days. In other words, **to take care of the truly sick.** Now, of course, it must take care of the entire population of "walking well" as well, a dramatically bigger contingent. Medicare was designed to take care of the truly ill, now it is charged to look for and search out any and all disease in the full population before symptoms even develop. A considerably more expensive task!

Also, there is the concept of first, second, and third day illness to appreciate. Walk-in clinics see a large volume of first day minor illnesses. Illnesses that would otherwise be gone in a day or two are seen in walk-in clinics because of ease of entry. It is often "runny nose medicine" that any granny could do. Frequently, physicians have to see patients who come to their offices hoping to prevent minor illness.

"Doc, I came in to see if I am going to get a sore throat... Bad time for me to be sick... A few in the office got it!"

"Oh..."

"Can I have some pills just to be sure, Doc?"

The nation cannot afford to continue this sort of mis-utilization when the patient as an individual definitely would not, if paying.

If a patient were not seen for these minor things in the first day, the great majority would not bother to come in the second day. They feel better. Likewise for second and third day waits. Progressively, they do not feel the need to come to the doctor. **This is the business of medicine. It is lucrative on the first day of minor complaints that are self-limiting. But Canada does not have enough money or health care human resources to deliver this kind of ineffective service.**

How can we continue to justify same day care for a cold and a six-month wait for treatment for can-

cer of the cervix?

Waiting lists are effectively 'soft caps' or controls on health service provision in a perverse way limiting utilization as I stated above. Unfortunately, the majority of wait time exists before secondary and tertiary specialty care or specialists' appointments, investigation and treatment, for generally the sickest people.

The only variant of these waiting lists is their length, the nature of the medical need and the service being waited for. In essence, then, **what kind of a wait list for which kind of service is acceptable?** Should it be measured only in time?

The public perception is that all patients on a wait list cannot and should not wait. After all, "They have time to die!"

Categorically, **there is no wait list for emergency services in Canada,** *yet.*

Reiterating, there is no wait list for emergencies such as heart attacks and broken legs, thanks to the doctors and nurses and allied health providers. They attempt to make sure the sickest get cared for first.

Patients must participate financially in their health costs if the system is ever to make sense and save dollars. Patient participation in the cost of their health care as a concept would naturally encourage the patient to take an active part in his or her wellness. Today, this is health care blasphemy.

What could be so wrong with this basic principle?
Would it deny service? No.

Would it reduce frivolous utilization? Yes, significantly.

Would it cause catastrophic personal costs? It would not have to.

Would it obligate up-front user fees? No, definitely not.

Again, if we have not defined the problem, then we are unlikely to find the correct solution.

Medicare is a wonderful and valuable social program, but it does not have even a semblance of the application of basic business principles and common sense.

What is wrong with prorated patient participation in the costs of health care?

What is wrong with something, anything, any measure whatsoever, on the demand side, to control frivolous utilization and ensure sustainability of our health care system?

CHAPTER 3

System Design

We need a sustainable affordable system suited to Canadians and their collective psyche.

I am not proposing chicken soup for the Canadian Health Care System, but I am suggesting that the consensus of all **those who do know and understand the current system is that it is good but *it is terminal.*** Like a tumour that outgrows its blood supply and as a result the tissue of its central part dies, the health system is outgrowing its money supply.

Mr. Romanow did not address the demand side at all, only the supply side. He had the opportunity to address the ills of the system, but he, in essence, recommended that we add more dollars to the current system and expand it. He **should have said to add more dollars *selectively*, increase the Federal component, and contract, not expand, the system.** Surely he did not really think any person or any advocacy group asked or consulted in Canada would advise the removal of resources. Of course not! They all said, "Give us more."

More money, more programs. Surprised?

As a past Premier, Mr. Romanow is fully aware of the fiscal brick wall that all provinces and territories are speeding down the track towards. Mr. Romanow and Mr. Kirby have both suggested that more cars be added to the train, that the train go faster, and that the track be somewhat lengthened. Unfortunately, with the same brick wall moved only slightly further down the line.

To add more financial resources, most, obviously, to be provided by the currently debt-ridden provinces, territories and the federal government, is a temporary solution. The medical analogy is to transfuse a hemorrhaging patient without bothering to first stop the hemorrhage. **Governments, if burdened further with even more debt and increased expectations, will hasten the health system's fiscal collapse and therefore do nothing for wellness or illness.**

Broadening the Medicare program to include the long-term care of everyone's parents will also hasten the health system's collapse. Care of one's parents, like the care of one's children, must be uniquely and primarily the responsibility of the family. If there is no family and no personal resources, then government should be involved partially or fully as a last resort. **Government participation as a last resort is basic Canadiana.** Taking care of those who cannot take care of themselves is a Canadian paradigm.

The acute part of our health care system must be preserved at all costs. I have used the word *acute*, not chronic or investigative, and not ongoing office monitoring of the walking well.

The high-level acute care system is considerably and increasingly more under-funded, but the overall health care system is adequately funded. I feel that even some parts are over-funded and deserve review.

Pyramid Comparisons

The shape of health care simplicity and sophistication is like a pyramid, naturally small on the top (sophisticated) and large on the bottom (simple) when referring to volume of services.

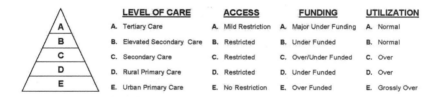

	LEVEL OF CARE	ACCESS	FUNDING	UTILIZATION
A	A. Tertiary Care	A. Mild Restriction	A. Major Under Funding	A. Normal
B	B. Elevated Secondary Care	B. Restricted	B. Under Funded	B. Normal
C	C. Secondary Care	C. Restricted	C. Over/Under Funded	C. Over
D	D. Rural Primary Care	D. Restricted	D. Under Funded	D. Over
E	E. Urban Primary Care	E. No Restriction	E. Over Funded	E. Grossly Over

Currently, **Canada in my estimation is financially under-funding the secondary and tertiary care systems.** This is creating a furor in our communities and amongst our hospital staffs, and with clear justification. **The primary care system is very arguably over-funded for the level of sophistication of what is being delivered and when it is being delivered.**

The furor in the primary care system is being fuelled, not by lack of funding, but by general lack of

physician availability and a lessening of good will on the part of the primary care providers to deliver comprehensive and all round continuing service to their practices as a collective.

For example, the large majority of Canadian patients, as a result of poor system design, have no after-hours alternative except to go to emergency rooms and walk-in clinics for non-emergent primary care. An emergency, in the eyes of the patient, is clearly different than in the eyes of a doctor.

There are three tender spots or common general complaints in our Canadian Health Care System that create the most public distress and upset:

- Firstly, no family doctor.

- Secondly, plugged emergency rooms.

- Thirdly, overrun of our elevated secondary and tertiary care systems, creating increasingly unreasonable waits and decreased access for the truly ill, both in our hospitals and at specialist providers' offices.

The Canadian Medicare System was originally designed for the 'truly ill' to alleviate and solve the third problem cited above and also to avoid catastrophic costs.

Supply of Family Doctors

The number one public complaint discussed

above is that some people have no family doctor.

We must look rationally at some elementary numbers and arithmetic:

About half of Canada's sixty thousand physicians are family doctors or general practitioners.

The Canadian Medical Association suggests that a good family practice size should average approximately sixteen to eighteen hundred patients.

If our thirty thousand primary care doctors were at the average patient load, that would add up to human resources capable of servicing forty-five to fifty million people or even more!

Canada's population is thirty-three million!

Adding or subtracting any fudge factors that one would wish, either doctors being semi-retired or with obligations to child raising or for whatever reason, we still should have ample family doctors.

Each province is correspondingly the same.

The territories, however, are suffering with considerably fewer than needed in all sectors.

Why do people not have a family doctor then?

Why is the office wait list for an appointment inordinately longer for secondary care or a specialist

than for a family doctor or for primary care?

I would like to suggest that it is a combination of several factors, such as the justifiable desire for an easier lifestyle,

too much referral to specialists of primary care work,

and high rotation of otherwise walking well patients in the primary care office.

There is no universal shortage of family doctors in Canada, just a shortage of service, availability and accountability, all as a result of a system poorly set up with yesterday's standards for today's world.

The answer for the person without a family doctor today is clearly not just to increase the production of family doctors but to properly utilize the current roster.

If doctors do not do the "doctoring" then who will? Society will soon find an alternate replacement. Indeed, this is what is occurring right now and frighteningly fast in primary care.

Crowded Emergency Rooms

The number two public complaint, plugged emergency rooms, is also largely a result of inappropriate over-utilization.

We are poorly designed in primary care; and inadequate after-hours servicing of primary care practices is largely the cardinal problem in our emergency rooms.

For instance, in the case of an emergency room in a region of twenty thousand people with fifteen family doctors working only days, how can one emergency room on-call doctor cover every practice after hours, Saturdays and Sundays? This is happening routinely across the country and is more the rule than the exception. As stated earlier, for many primary care physicians, at six p.m. each day and on weekends their patients become the government's patients and some patients are even told this.

Poor Access for the Very Ill

Our public acrimony number three: decreased access for the truly ill, is far more serious and has far more important implications for our future demographic medical needs.

The patients at this level of medical need are truly ill and have to have rapid comprehensive care. Care for cancer, cardiac events, trauma and so on must be available and expedient.

As you may perceive, the pyramid of care I conceptually diagrammed above is based only on the number and sophistication of services. There are a large amount of minor services and a small amount of major services.

If one were to look at the degree of or the severity of illness and the absolute need for care, then the pyramid would be upside down.

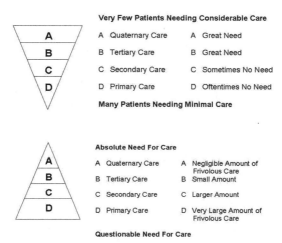

Very Few Patients Needing Considerable Care

A Quaternary Care	A Great Need
B Tertiary Care	B Great Need
C Secondary Care	C Sometimes No Need
D Primary Care	D Oftentimes No Need

Many Patients Needing Minimal Care

Absolute Need For Care

A Quaternary Care	A Negligible Amount of Frivolous Care
B Tertiary Care	B Small Amount
C Secondary Care	C Larger Amount
D Primary Care	D Very Large Amount of Frivolous Care

Questionable Need For Care

The pyramid of nonsense and frivolous utilization consuming our health system, on the other hand, is right side up, the most frivolous care being located in primary care.

Over Utilization

Most of the frivolous use of health resources is in primary care.

There is also a large amount in secondary care.

Obviously, not too many people overuse quaternary care, such as brain surgery or coronary by-pass surgery.

The human resource need or need for doctors is an inverse pyramid. Generally, the higher the level of care given by the provider, the bigger the shortage throughout the system.

However, some disciplines in secondary care are over-populated with doctors and are over-servicing. Secondary care is a mixed bag of frivolous over-service and true under-service. This also includes too much primary care being done more expensively by secondary care physicians.

There is also much marginally useless procedural medicine being done with very low yield or scientific justification and it is very costly.

We do not have much data on the efficacy of some services, the yield, or the medical outcomes of many procedures. For instance, when should knee arthroscopy for pain be done? Should it be done at all if we have adequate MRI availability that sometimes is a better diagnostic alternative? The fee moves from orthopedics to radiology. Certainly, the medical risk becomes nearly zero with MRI versus arthroscopy.

For the amount of money it consumes, we must do a better job in health care and only do the medical things that need to be done.

But how?

Simply put, we need data and we also need patient participation in the financial process to control utilization.

Control on demand side.

Now again, that is blasphemy! Right! What a horror!

Patients may have to contribute financially on an individual basis.

They may also have to be told that they do not need a service.

The sicker the patient, the higher the level of care and therefore, costs.

Expansion of certain sectors of our health system should occur and contraction of other parts should be more clearly defined and carried out.

A National Plan

So what shape should the new pyramid of physician-patient care take on?
Should it be a pyramid? Maybe not.
Which part needs broadening and which part needs narrowing?

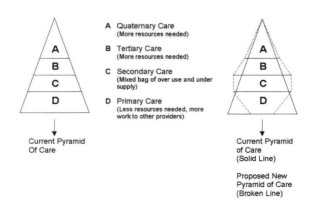

A Quaternary Care
(More resources needed)

B Tertiary Care
(More resources needed)

C Secondary Care
(Mixed bag of over use and under supply)

D Primary Care
(Less resources needed, more work to other providers)

Current Pyramid
Of Care

Current Pyramid
of Care
(Solid Line)

Proposed New
Pyramid of Care
(Broken Line)

Where should other providers fit in?
We need more specialists and financial re-sources in quaternary care, tertiary care and some selected specialties in secondary care.

We need fewer primary care doctors and more cost efficient alternative human resource choices in primary care.

New medical graduates are now voting on primary care with their feet by not going into primary care. Fewer medical graduates now want to do primary care, whatever that is today, and whatever it is going to be tomorrow. **Our family practice residency training seats in Canada last year were not all filled.**

A large majority of primary care doctors, now mostly in larger urban areas, get remunerated far too much for the sophistication of what they do and for the things they do not do. Why do fewer of our medical school grads want to take up primary care?

If we are to advise more changes to our health care system, we should be reflective of the patterns of change that have taken place over the last thirty years. The direction of momentum must be observed and written into any future plan. Mr. Romanow has suggested, as cited above, to simply move the fiscal wall further down the track. We will still surely hit it! He has not suggested any basic system design adjustment or change. As Gary Mar, Minister of Health for Alberta has said in many speeches, "The only change people do not resist is a diaper change."

Demand Side Control

Mr. Romanow has suggested that more account-ability measures be applied to the provinces by the federal government. But the provinces put in eighty-five percent of the costs, and mandatory provincial accounting for the remaining fifteen percent of federal money received seems to be rather moot.

It is overtly elementary that **it is not territorial, provincial or federal accountability that Canada's Health Care System needs.** Heaven forbid! **It is accountability on the part of the patients and providers at the provision consumption interface level that is needed.** There is virtually no accountability there now and Mr. Romanow has not suggested any.

The idea that every health service provided in Canada is an absolutely necessary service is ridiculous. A vast number of health care services provided in Canada today, if not done at all, would make no difference at all. Usually, this is service delivered lower down on the therapeutic ladder of care.

If we are to have a national health care system, then we need a national approach and a consentual plan. Thirteen plans will not work. Why should a visit to a doctor for an ear infection be paid out with less than twenty dollars in Newfoundland and nearly twice that elsewhere?

We have had the Romanow Report, the National Health Care Forum, the Mazinkowski Report, the Fyke Report, the Kirby Report and a partridge in a pear tree.

We are probably no further ahead.

When there are many and diverse opinions on the solution to a problem, then chances are that none is correct or the problem has not really been properly defined.

Report after report by governments has delayed remedial action and deferred political decisions for governments. The process initially excites and subsequently disappoints the people. "Another moon walk report," appearing to go forward when actually standing still or going backward.

Illness care compared to wellness initiatives is consuming too much of our tax resources, proportionately.

Fortunately, we are almost all born with good health. Very small numbers of Canadian babies have anything but excellent health and they all possess brand new body systems. Aging and the things we do subsequently to ourselves mitigate against our health. We (society) eat poorly, we eat too much, we do not exercise enough, we smoke too much, we drink too much alcohol, we use too much medication, we do not value the traditional family, and we use too much illicit drugs.

We are born, unfortunately, with no education, which has to be imparted by society. **Good health is a product of and follows good education.**

Good education generally leads to good em-

ployment and lifestyle and those are the major determinants of good health, both on a societal basis and
on an individual basis.

The Canadian people should put education as
their number one priority and health will follow.

The financial attention paid to each should parallel this position. It will result in both better education and better health down the road and better
wellness en route.

We are currently enjoying living in very good financial times. **If we have an economic down turn and increasing interest rates in Canada, our social programs,
especially health, will become even more precarious.**
We should be prepared.

CHAPTER 4

Prorated Patient Participation

A large percentage of Canadian people have said that they would gladly pay more tax to sustain their Medicare system.

The Romanow Report does not suggest that patients participate in their costs of health care, but supports a singular public system. Mr. Romanow has suggested that governments should put in more money and that the system should remain publicly funded. I agree to a degree. However, **governments have stated clearly that they cannot afford the current expenditures, let alone the projected expenditures.** The question arises then, as to where the extra money should come from or whom the money should come from, and how it should be collected.

The extra money that the system is craving may all come from the proposed "private patient sector" or the high earners.

This would create two clear divisions of health care.

A private system for those who are able to pay and a public system for the remainder: *duality.*

It is graphically illustrated below.

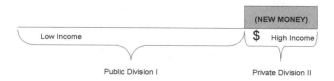

Or the new money could come from a tax-based prorated patient participation process true to the Canadian spirit.

Every health care consumer would contribute something, but those who could pay more, would pay more, based on their ability to pay; it would be a tax-based system.

For instance, a patient with a very low taxable income, below a chosen figure, would pay nothing. A patient with a very high income would pay a certain amount, and all in between would pay a varying graduated or prorated amount. Patients would have their own prorated maximum cost above which government would pay all.

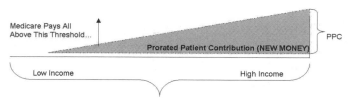

There would be no duality and only one tier. This is what most Canadians seem to want. We are awaiting the word of the Supreme Court of Canada in mid-2004 on just this issue, the legality of private health care.

Clearly, if any accountability is to be applied to patients and doctors, then continuing the current "no cost to the patient, no accountability for the doctor" system is mindless. A waiting and indignant elderly patient once said to me, "Why should I walk every day and take care of myself well, as I did all my life, and subsidize those louts who don't give a damn about their health and cost the system a fortune?" Rather simplistically profound, I thought.

If one were to ask most Canadians if they would accept a system of partial patient payment, for example a ninety/ten percent split, or risk the total collapse of the one hundred percent system, the answer would be a clear "yes".

Notice that I have not used anywhere in the text the two health-care "four letter words", *user* and *fees*.

Emphatically, **there would be no up-front fees based on use. No cash. No cheques. No credit cards. No debit cards. And no denial of service for the sake of money. Only a tax-based system, very much akin to our RRSP system.**

There would be a system of prorated patient participation in the cost of their care. It is called *accountability* and has been categorically avoided by all health studies and reports to date.

Maintaining the Principles of Medicare

There are two cardinal provisos or basic principles of Medicare that have to be absolutely protected if we move to a prorated patient participation system:

- **Number one: No financial restriction to access the system for anyone.**
- **Number two: Protection from catastrophic costs for everyone.**

Developing a system of prorated patient participation in costs that has these provisions built in would be a major paradigm shift in the Canadian Health Care System psychology. It would have to be agreed upon by all jurisdictions and carried out by all at the same time.

One would have to take care of one's health or pay some prorated price. Those born with, affected by, or inflicted with major life-long health problems would be protected as well.

Any health care system without user and provider accountability is abused, as ours clearly is.

The federal government's position on provincial and territorial accountability for spending in health is irrelevant considering nearly half of provincial-territorial spending goes to health.

Why not do it? Why not have patients participate financially in their health care in a prorated fashion?

➤ Prorated patient participation in costs of their care would still allow for complete accessibility.

➤ Prorated patient participation would significantly reduce utilization and prevent duality, or two unequal systems, one for most and the other for a few.

➤ Cost control and continued quality assurance would become intrinsic to the system. Horse sense instead of always more dollars for a remedy.

➤ Patient participation would address sustainability more assuredly than just more money on the supply side and nothing on the demand side.

➤ More money, more programs and no real intent to restructure the system with a plan or a design would only defer the problem to another report, study or commission or whatever down the political road.

Health care reform to date has been more about health care re-infrastructuring than health care restructuring.

Mr. Romanow is a little bit correct for the political health-care present, but very much wrong for the future sustainability of our Canadian Health Care System. Mr. Romanow delivered the report and disappeared. "Who was that masked man?" Who is left behind, designated to do what has to be done? Who is in charge? Who is responsible? Who will coordinate the re-tooling and re-gearing of the thirteen health care jurisdictions?

**The Romanow Report avoided the major issue
of affordability and cost containment!**

CHAPTER 5

Doctors

The solicitous reader may question what has happened with doctors in the past forty years since Medicare began.

What has transpired since doctors at the beginning of Medicare resisted Medicare by going on strike in Saskatchewan?

What has happened since the number of doctors in Canada has more than doubled over these years, relative to population?

What has happened since the percentage of GDP spending on health care has gone from seven to ten percent?

What has happened since the specialist doctor registration, a small fraction of the total number of doctors registered forty years ago, now equals general practitioners?

What has happened since the medical school entrants were essentially all male compared to the present day when forty-four percent or so are male and fifty-six percent are female?

What has happened over the last several decades since the population of Canada has increased by twenty-five percent and the population of physicians by over one hundred percent?

Fittingly, and because I am one as well, I will talk about medical doctors initially, considering they are on the top of the patient's therapeutic ladder.

There is a therapeutic ladder concept in health care.

The upper part of the ladder is care for patients who are very sick, and their intensive care is provided by very highly trained professionals, usually specialist doctors. Of course the less sick the patient, the less trained the physician, specialist or professional, has to be.

The continuum goes on down the ladder through all the different health professionals, with much overlapping, to simple care inevitably done by the patient himself or herself or by a parent.

The ladder is getting longer as the science of health care advances and doctors become even more specialized. It is continuously lengthening because of the modern progress of health care sophistication and because of increasing needs demanding a provider higher and more qualified on the ladder. For instance, from Granny, who may put on a band aid, to the licensed practical nurse, to the nurse, to the family doctor, to the cardiovascular surgeon or brain surgeon.

The Demise of the General Practitioner

Over the years in my work in health care, I have had the benefit of knowing and working with many doctors who practiced prior to Medicare. Their jobs were vocations. For the most part, they were very devoted and ever available for ministering their profession. They competed professionally with each other; the physician across the street or down the road was a colleague but also a competitor. They were happy, and eager, to see any patient walk into their office for service.

Patients were solicitous and fearful of cost. They asked doctors to do as much as possible locally and for as little cost as possible. They were paying! They did not want to, nor could they miss work.

Most physicians were extremely fortunate when they received fifty percent of accounts receivable. Many times, payment was only a solemn promise of gifts of food: sometimes a chicken, and sometimes vegetables were the order of the day.

After-hours, on-call rosters for doctors were unusual. They were all on call virtually all the time. General practitioners usually "came in" to the hospital emergency room or the hospital wards themselves, anytime, for their patients in order to keep them. Each general practitioner usually did "his" own deliveries.

I estimate that ninety percent of health care was delivered by general practitioners prior to Medicare. There were half as many doctors at that time, very hungry for work, with essentially the same Canadian population. What has happened? A physician whom I know well practiced prior to Medicare. He related to me once that in the seventies they frequently used to say before Medicare arrived, "If you think that medical care is expensive now, wait until it is free."

Certainly, compared to today, a broad medical knowledge base was needed by general practitioners, and extremely sensitive and acute diagnostic clinical ability in the absence of today's quality investigative tools. Today, each physician group has a relatively more concentrated knowledge base. Largely, clinical skills have been replaced by technological investigation, both laboratory and diagnostic imaging.

Jokingly, many GP's would relate, "Was the neurological consult report CAT scan positive or CAT scan negative?" Indeed, today's patients ask for, believe in, and largely trust technology, or the "pan man scan", more than their doctor. Laboratories and diagnostic imaging techniques now make the lion's share of the diagnoses. Clinical diagnosis is more and more rare. "Rare like rocking horse dung," an instructor once told me.

Another senior physician friend, who was forty years in the profession, once said to me a long time ago, "If they are sick, give 'em pills, if they are neurotic, give 'em tests but give 'em something! Keep them moving!" I tend to believe mostly everybody gets both today, whether they need it or not, regardless of price. Or should I say ignorant of price?

Then what really has changed and why? Forty years ago, there were general practitioners and a very small number of consultants or specialists. There were, in essence, two general groups of specialists: surgeons and internal medicine specialists. Basically, the only hospital-based doctors were radiologists and pathologists.

Surgeons were further subdivided into "head" specialists, chest, brain and general surgeons. General practitioners did most anesthesias.

In very large centers, the sub-specialties in both medicine and surgery were evolving rapidly, along with the bulk of knowledge that needed to be known by each. Specialties such as orthopedics, gynecology, pediatrics, cardiology, and so on were evolving. Soon the sections or divisions of care were called primary care, secondary care and eventually tertiary care. Now we have what qualifies as quaternary care; that is, care even more sophisticated and higher than third level care.

Primary care is provided by doctors who work in their offices, public clinics or walk-in clinics, and do mostly non-urgent and non-emergent medical care and follow-up.

Secondary care is given usually by specialists and sometimes by general practitioners. It is a higher level of care such as general surgery, internal medicine, some uncomplicated anesthesia, obstetrics, pediatrics, some routine orthopedic fractures and the like.

Tertiary care, or a third level of doctors, do even more specialized and more complicated care such as brain surgery, open heart surgery, complicated anesthesia, cancer care and the like.

Quaternary care is given by even more specialized doctors, doing such things as pediatric neuro surgery, pediatric cardiac surgery, pediatric or infant cancer, and many other highly sophisticated procedures and investigations done by highly and selectively trained professionals.

The nature of physician services has changed dramatically because the nature of patient expectation and demand has changed even more dramatically.

The general practitioner of some years ago did a large volume of a little bit of everything. At the time, "he" was expected to be a multi and mini-specialist doing the lion's share of the work. The general practitioner did cardiology, pediatrics, radiology, obstetrics, some general surgery, scopes, anesthesia, orthopedics, gynecology, psychiatry, trauma, oncology and anything more that appeared and had to be done, even dentistry. There was nobody else, and transportation to other caregivers was difficult, often distant and frowned upon. Referral was often seen as a professional failure.

The Role of Medical Schools

Twenty-five years ago, we agreed to change the face of general practice. I remember clearly, at the time, the medical training establishment saying that we needed to train an enhanced general practitioner. A super general practitioner, a specialist generalist!

A whole new set of professors in their own family practice "specialty" was needed in all medical schools, the traditional domain of specialists. It was decided to add another year to general practice internship, call it a residency; and then the better-trained new graduate doctor would be capable of doing much more. For instance, it was purported that the new general practitioner could do caesarean sections, forceps deliveries, some scopes, anesthesia and so on. They would be capable of more sophisticated medicine, surgery, radiology, psychiatry, pediatrics and emergency medicine. They could work in rural areas with confidence having had this broader in-depth training and experience. They would be called family doctors, as opposed to general practitioners, whatever that means, and have a national certification.

There is corridor discussion now about reversing this decision. I believe it needs review.

It has been more than twenty years since this change happened and I, and many like me, still do not understand! Much the reverse of what was intended has unfortunately occurred. Firstly, we lost one full graduate year. Secondly, the modern family doctor's training virtually relegates the new trainee to large metropolitan city office medicine. For the most part, the additional training has been far less experiential and almost precludes working in small towns, some cities and remote rural locations on one's own!

In the decision making process for the new graduate during medical training, the buck has always stopped with someone else. On graduation, it stops with the graduate, especially in rural Canada. In rural Canada, the family doctor is very much on his or her own with little or no specialist backup. In urban Canada's larger cities, specialists are immediately available to help family doctors when a medical situation warrants.

Some medical schools have made the effort to have curricula that help guide graduates towards more rural and remote practice. Bravo *Memorial* and *Sherbrooke* who have made a good effort.

Indeed **over the last few years, medical school grads have been avoiding family practice residency as a trend and are more frequently selecting specialty residencies instead.** Why not? Two more years gives a specialty. "You have to be a specialist today to be a "real doctor", said one of my vintage general practitioner colleagues some years ago. He went on to say that most of the new grads today are like allied health professionals with prescription pads. This is a sad commentary.

Just recently a leader in the Canadian medical establishment said publicly that you had to work in a rural area to be a "real doctor". What does that make newly trained urban family doctors? Urbane?

As we watch and listen incessantly about primary care reform, what we once knew as primary care provided by the general practitioner or the discipline of general practice is quite clearly disappearing. Primary care is best explained as the care done for patients on entry to the health system by general practitioners or family doctors.

I do not like the connotation of the word "reform" suggesting something is and was wrong with what general practitioners used to do and currently do in most situations. Health care is changing and we must change with it. I like the concept of primary care innovation.

Doctors in training are becoming uninterested in primary care, are not challenged professionally by their new lot in family medicine and are not very interested in being in rural Canada. The up-migration of primary care medical work to secondary care providers' (specialists') hands has been rapid and huge. The down-migration of primary care to the hands of alternative care providers has also been large and insidious.

Alternative care providers are best described as non-physician health care people who now do many things once only done by family doctors. It is said that sixty percent of people seek advice from one sort or another of alternative care provider. Inevitably, they seek and are getting considerably more time with the alternative care provider than with their physician, and are happy to pay.

The family doctors and general practitioners of today rarely do deliveries, hence mid-wives;

reluctantly do emergency coverage, hence emergentologists;

reluctantly do on-call and hospital work, hence hospitalists.

Hospitalists are family doctors who work only in hospitals on salary usually to take care of other family doctors' patients when those family doctors prefer not to take care of hospital patients.

Family doctors rarely and reluctantly do concentrated care unit work, hence intensivists.

Intensivists are doctors who take care of family doctors' patients who are in intensive care units.

And lastly, in many circumstances for no practical reasons, family doctors refuse to take new patients, hence the movement towards nurse practitioners and other alternative providers.

We must understand clearly the reasons for these changes before we attempt to 'reform' or 'innovate' primary care.

Primary Care Innovation

The solo general practitioner is nearly gone. Some left solo practice reluctantly and some left by choice. Some hang on, I am one. The multi-disciplinary family medicine team and center is nearly here. Patients will relate to a family medicine place, not to a doctor. This concept is not new. It was here thirty years ago.

We need to move as many full-scope-practice nurses and allied health providers into primary care teams as soon as possible. This is the story of primary care innovation needed.

If we recruit the projected need for specialist people from within the family doctor system, then the process of producing a specialist will be virtually cut in half. If we use technicians in the system where the procedure is rote and purely technical, we will reduce the need for physicians and other professionals in short supply. **If we do not, we will wake up in 2010 with some major medical services unavailable where they exist now in various Canadian hospital units.**

If this need is not addressed soon, then pressure will be loaded upon high-level acute care with such intensity that it will pale the currently alleged need for more family doctors.

The Health Council of Canada

Who is in charge?

Who will make these necessary changes? Even a squirrel has enough wisdom to prepare for winter.

Will it be Mr. Romanow's proposed new Health Council of Canada?

Will it have any jurisdiction?

Will it have any power?
I hope so, but I expect not.

It appears, as some have already voiced, that the Health Council of Canada that Mr. Romanow has suggested may be ineffective because it has not been empowered.

Jurisdiction in health is currently fully provincial-territorial; and given that the federal financial component is less than fifteen percent, clearly the provincial-territorial capitals of Canada may take suggestions but not take direction from such an agency.

Alberta is not attending and Quebec is usually non-participatory.

An agency such as that does not have responsibility for public spending or cost control.

The proposed Health Council of Canada may, however, be a very good candidate to advocate for limits on the demand side. Now *there* is a very interesting and novel concept. All governments would like to have that happen and blame someone else.

There has been a large booming quiet since the Romanow Report. Who is following up? The departments of health of Canada cannot be expected to juggle and sweep the floor at the same time.

We cannot continue, without a plan, to depend on the graduates of foreign medical schools. This is an uncertain resource where the quality of training is difficult to assess and with various other difficulties aside from medicine to be managed. We need a formal system for assessing the further training needed for foreign trained physicians for certification in Canada. (Mr. Romanow has this issue correct, recommendation forty-seven.)

We now have a health system in Canada that is very rapidly selecting and separating out our hospital-based (real doctors) and office-based (presumably unreal doctors).

Then there are the "real" rural doctors. These are doctors who do full scope practice and continue to be both hospital and office-based. They tend to be older. There are fewer of these doctors now by virtue of age, and because of the apparently inadequate training of new graduates for rural medicine in all round general practice. The rural general practitioner has to be a mini-specialist in every discipline. The new primary care graduates do not seem to have the training or the appetite necessary to work in rural Canada. Neither do they get the opportunity to gain adequate practical experience during training to do so. The desire to work and live in rural Canada is becoming more rare.

Quick Fixes

General practitioners and family doctors have tacitly accepted "walk-in" clinics.

Walk-in clinics are known as hit and run "Mac-medicine" with pitifully little, if any, follow-up or continuity.

Of course this is mostly because private practices that used to be traditionally covered after hours are now for the most part not.

Most family doctors or general practitioners will agree that walk-in clinics have diluted quality, disillusioned patients, and created an atmosphere of abrogation on the part of the walk-in clinic physician and inequity among medical providers.

Walk-in clinics have magnified what I call "one hand" medicine, the other hand being firmly placed on the door-knob of the exam room. This has led to a quiet clandes-tine conflict between the idealistically motivated general practitioner and those motivated by money alone. I dis-agree with the walk-in clinic movement. **Walk-in clinic visits should be paid substantially less than regular office visits.**

I saw a patient not too long ago in the late nine-teen-nineties.
Patient: "Hi, Doc."
Me: "Hi, what can I do for you?"
Patient: "I saw Doctor so and so this morning."
Me: "What do you need?"
Patient: "Well, I was in the walk-in clinic... this morn-ing... He came in... he didn't look at me... musta been rushed... Poor guy... He picked up a tongue depressor... stuck it in my mouth as I was starting to sit down... I couldn't talk then... he took it out... by that time I was sitting quietly down... He was busy writing a prescription... I waited... He left abruptly without looking at me."

Me: "So, what can I do for you?"
Patient: "My throat's not sore, Doc. It's my back!"
Unfortunately humorous, *true* and in its own way,
tragic.

The flow-through of office-based patients in primary
care is also quite rapid and simple. The large majority of
the office-based patients seen by family doctors are either
A – Treated as prescribed by a specialist's consult,
or
B – If significantly ill, are sent to an emergency room
to another doctor, or
C – If the complaint is of a minor nature, they are
treated there, or
D – If the complaint seems simple and is undiag-
nosed, they are sent for investigation.

Counseling and disease education is becoming
more a rarity because of the overall basic flaws in the system. It is hard to believe that primary care reform, or *innovation* as I like to call it, is as ill defined as it is.

We must ascertain and reveal the reasons for the
increasingly higher price paid for less and less sophisticated medical care delivered in a family doctor's medical
office from nine to five, five days a week.

Back to Full Scope

**General practitioners and family doctors can-
not continue en mass to retreat only to office hours
five days per week.** In very many cases, after-hours coverage by general practitioners of family practices is not

arranged. Clearly, **patients have health care problems twenty-four hours a day, seven days a week.** This, then, results in fewer rungs on the lower end of the therapeutic ladder for many general practitioners and family doctors. **This situation also results in unbearable loads of non-emergency patients in our emergency rooms after regular daytime hours and on weekends.** It appears that many doctors feel that when they are finished at the business day's end, the patient becomes the government's problem.

Family doctors have to get back to doing "full scope or all round general practice".

This means full scope in service and full scope around the clock and the week, twenty-four seven.

Nurses want full scope practice and it seems family doctors do not.

To date, full scope all round general practice is more common and more preserved in rural areas and seems to have survived in the rural areas out of necessity. General practitioners in rural areas and relatively small cities still do in-hospital care such as obstetrics, emergency room coverage, hospital on-call, some fractures, acute cardiac care and pediatrics. They have no other choice but to leave the area where they work or to stay for altruistic reasons.

Family doctors who practice in rural Canada have now further defined themselves as different. They have their own association, meetings and a national journal!

However, there still is an increasingly difficult challenge to recruit new graduates, who seem ill prepared to go to rural practice situations. There are many reasons for this. Inadequate preparation is one reason as stated, and lifestyle is another.

Canada needs to redesign and reform the face of medical care delivery pertaining to doctors and their health care colleagues. We need a national strategy and a long-term plan.

Although eighty percent of the Canadian population lives in cities with populations larger than ten thousand people, six million or more of us still live in rural Canada. **The provider needs to be trained to suit the Canadian system, not the converse.**

The therapeutic ladder I referred to above, once having ninety percent of the rungs occupied by the general practice doctor group, is for the most part now starting to have fewer if any rungs left on it for general practitioners or family doctors. There are even fewer rungs on the ladder in large urban centers though today's therapeutic ladder is conceptually much longer than it was twenty-five years ago.

The passive migration of primary care services to the much more expensive secondary care provider is called referral or specialist consultation. This factor is extremely significant and much is largely unjustifiable.

Referral or consultation appears to be higher in urban than in rural areas and may be between thirty and fifty percent for some primary care doctors. **The continued attempt to speed up patient flow in fee-for-service general practice is driving this phenomenon.** As a result, there are even fewer upper rungs on the therapeutic ladder for general practitioners, as specialists do more and more family doctor work by virtue of abrogation, and of course this is increasing the pressure on specialists. Also **as a result, there are long waiting lists for specialists.**

Nurse practitioners, on the other hand, **are claiming quite vocally and validly that they can do three quarters of the office practice work of general practitioners and family doctors.** They claim fiercely that they want to improve the situation for the patients by "spending more time", "doing more teaching", "adding more care to primary care", and "allowing patients with no family doctor to be cared for". Obviously, they also claim they will "do it for less money". Alarmingly, **this proposal sounds like what family doctors are not doing and should be doing to infuse confidence and satisfaction back into the doctor-patient-government relationship.**

Changing Roles of Providers

Storefront or walk-in alternative primary health care today is exploding in capability, capacity and diversity. Psychologists, physiotherapists, massage therapists, sports medicine people, optometrists and many others are doing traditional general practice also and as well as the general practitioner.

General practitioners and family doctors are now edging slowly but surely towards being an expensive redundancy. They seem to be over-trained for the work they do in urban areas and under-trained for the work that is needed in rural areas. Considering the abrogation factors mentioned above, and with primary care referral rates as high as fifty percent in some practices; and with a compulsory system of referral to see a specialist, *we must question the real need for more family doctors.* **Possibly we need increased production of specialists with direct patient access without referral to the specialty service.** A good question I feel needs to be addressed.

The "gate theory" of primary care, which theoretically is supposed to protect secondary care from frivolous over-utilization, has obviously not held up to scrutiny. I think it is actually making the specialists' lives worse. **In effect, today's multi-specialist system of secondary care and higher care is yesterday's general practice system.**

This factor no doubt has increased the quality and intensity of care for the truly ill, but what will be the future of the family doctor and general practitioner? Will they be captains of multi-disciplinary teams? Physician assistants? How will they be paid? How much will they be paid? How much training do they really need? Can someone else do it?

I suspect family doctors are moving insidiously, unknowingly and with much denial towards self-propagated obsolescence.

Is a family doctor with only eight hundred or one thousand patients, who works thirty-six hours a week, who never does a delivery, never fixes a fracture, never takes care of a hospital patient, never works in an emergency room, and never assists in the operating room a real doctor? Another good question.

On how many occasions have physicians, myself included, been introduced as a medical doctor only to be followed by the statement: "Nice to meet you. Are you a specialist or 'just a general practitioner?'" I suspect that before long the comment "just a general practitioner" may be justified. Any labor union person could give our Canadian general practitioners and family doctors a lesson in not giving away one's work! It will most certainly soon be done by someone else, and one will be out of a job.

The role of the general practitioner and family doctor must be rethought.

Health care is not eight hours a day and must be given by the right person, at the right time, in the right location and for the right price.

Should we pay the appropriate price for the service or pay for the qualifications of the service provider regardless of the simplicity of the service? This is another very salient question.

General practitioners and family doctors are frequently giving care and are frequently required to give care that is largely unnecessary.

In turn, **specialists are doing a large volume of primary care instead of only secondary care.** This is obviously very needlessly expensive to the system.

Society holds doctors in great esteem and accords them very high stature. Their expectations and incomes are consistent with this esteem. **This will not continue into the future for the walk-in clinic doctor and the office-based forty-hour or less a week physician with no after business hours coverage of their patients.**

Today many patients are well educated and oftentimes do not need any health care provider. Self-management of disease is common. For instance, glucometers, pregnancy tests, spirometers, automated blood pressure monitors and more were not available twenty-five years ago and today are common.

My eighty-five year old mother, God bless her, took her own blood pressure and pulse religiously every day. One day her pulse was thirty-five instead of the usual seventy and her pressure was different. She called the emergency room, explained, and the diagnosis of third-degree heart block was made on the phone. "Come in, Missus, you may need a pacemaker." She did need a pacemaker!

This results in less need of the primary care physician. Then where does the public clamor and claim of a physician shortage and the reality of all the incessant demand for utilization come from? Good question!

Medical schools are going on blithely training medical doctors for whatever the trainee medical doctor wants to train for, not what the system needs. We have a virtual schism between Canadian ministries of health and the Association of Canadian Medical Colleges or our medical schools. They do not talk and they do not meet. **This is a critical weakness in the Canadian system.** There is not and has not been any meaningful communication between the widget user, so to speak, and the widget maker. Health dollars are being spent with no attention being paid to health "sense".

Again, we need a national consensus and plan for the immediate and distant future for medical human resources.

In 1992, we shut down ten percent of our medical school seats as a result of the Barer-Stoddart Report. Almost at the same time, we lost a graduation year due to the doubling of general practitioner post-grad training to produce the super general practitioners or the new "family doctors". These moves were made for cost control. It was thought that limiting the number of doctors, limiting the number of beds, limiting the wages that could be earned, limiting the number of nurses; installing ceilings of all and sundry sorts would control costs. **These moves did not control costs and produced immense provider and consumer frustration.**

Historically, all cost containment moves seem to have been applied to the provider side of the health care triangle. After working in and with the health care system for over thirty years, I cannot remember any substantial cost containment maneuvers applied

with any gusto to the consumer side of the health care triangle. There is never anything to control the demand side, utilization. Again, patients are voters.

Boomer Demographics

The "graying" of the medical profession has obviously been an aggravating factor in the situation as well. The baby boomer population effect has concurrently affected and stressed the doctor population as well as others, and has created supply and demand inequities. Older doctors naturally can only work less and wish to work less. They have this right but not this privilege today in many circumstances.

Younger doctors in search of a better lifestyle do not seem to want extended hours in general. They want contracted hours and expanded pay. The effect is compounded by a great increase in demand for service by the patients.

My impression, that I express with some peril here, is that **the gender neutralization of the medical profession that has happened recently has increased the number of grads that are female but decreased service availability of the whole cohort.** Based on an average fifty-hour workweek, males work an average of about fifty-seven hours and females about forty-three hours.

Then where do we go from here? **A comprehensive medical and health human-resource plan for Canada is clearly a must.** It must address the questions and observations expressed above, and more: the right kind of provider, in the right location, with the right training, at the right cost, with continuous system monitoring and analysis. It must involve all the proponents and providers; certainly the medical schools at least should be involved.

In 2015, we will have started peaking out on the needs of the baby boomers. The peak of the load of boomers will be about fifty-five years old at that time. Theoretically, we will not need as many doctors thereafter. Heaven forbid that we make the same error as in 1992, only in reverse.

Ontario is in the process of building a new medical school based in Sudbury and Thunder Bay humorously called "Thunderbury". It will start turning out new grads just about when we should be thinking about rationalizing our numbers again because of reduced need at the peak and subsequent reduction of the number of high-health-consuming baby boomers.

Because of over production of physicians, some countries in Europe have experienced many doctors driving taxis! The OECD countries have an average of 2.9 physicians per thousand people. Canada has 2.1 per thousand. The USA has 2.8. Italy certainly skews the average with 6 doctors per thousand people.

In other words, **Canada has one doctor for approximately every four hundred and seventy people.**

The supply of and the demand for physicians is a dynamic and an elusive target at best. Obviously, it depends on utilization, either open-ended or controlled. Also, it depends on the nature of the physician. This factor is largely underestimated by all in the system today. What services are physicians adequately trained for and able to provide, and which services do they want to do? When is the physician willing to provide these services, and where is a physician willing to provide these services? Simplistic, but actually much of the root of the problem. Why should a patient knowingly see a doctor who cannot care for the existing problem only to get referred to another one who is capable or wants to give the care? Expensive business. It would not happen in the private sector.

We now have an asymmetry between what patients want for service and what service physicians are willing to provide, and when physicians are willing to provide the service. We are seeing a growing gap between the price that physicians expect for services rendered and the cost value placed on these services by governments and some taxpayers. Currently, the dollar value for a health service provided is being questioned, more now than ever, especially in primary care or at the family doctor level. Walk-in clinic fees are an example.

Open-ended utilization, amongst other things, is magnifying the alleged and relative shortage of family doctors, and this factor is driving the costs of physician services at the negotiating tables.

Canada has approximately thirty thousand active general practitioners and family doctors, as stated above.

A practice size for primary care of sixteen to eighteen hundred patients is what the Canadian Medical Association recommends.

That gives coverage for forty-five to fifty million Canadians.

Everyone knows there are thirty-three million Canadians.

Where is the primary care shortage?

Why do some Canadians not have a family doctor?

CHAPTER 6

Nurses

Florence Nightingale, a British aristocrat and an un-likely personal-care attendant at the time, was the first nurse to apply science to nursing. She went to the Crimean War front and applied new hygienic techniques to wound care.

She was the so-called first "trained nurse" and trained the first of Canada's "trained nurses". Mostly they worked in hospital health and later in public and community health.

"I rang the bell, Doctor, but she didn't come!" A refrain I heard incessantly years ago. Patients had a perception that it was the responsibility of the nurse on duty to respond to every call from everybody.

"What did you need? Were you sick or in distress?" I would respond.

"No, Doctor, I needed my bed adjusted."

"Why did you not get out of bed and do it yourself? It would be good for you to stay active."

"Well, Doctor, I was too tired and the nurses are

here for that!"
"Why argue," I would muse.

This was a frequent interchange and probably a fair indicator of some inherent problems in our system since Medicare. Today we have self operated electric beds.

We are spoiled now. All and every service is expected right away and with a nursing smile; the patient, also with a resultant smile, expects no charge, better than at home!

The Canadian nurse, along with all other health providers, has also an extremely large respect in our society, probably because they answered ninety-nine percent of all bells! The one percent missed was probably because the nurse, he or she now, was answering another bell.

Queen Victoria's Victorian Order of Nurses, the VON, were the so-called first nurse practitioners, who did the lion's share of the work in public health and community health in early Canada.

The role of the Victorian Order of Nurses has now changed significantly. Once very large in public health and hospital care, they are now relegated to other sorts of private nursing such as home care or private immunization needs.

Background

In the early days, nurses were generically untrained females who did personal care. Then, sometime later, they were called "trained nurses", or nurses who had formal training in doing patient care. Subsequently, we saw nurses "registered" after two, sometimes three, years of formal in-service training in a hospital milieu, now called RN's. Now, with a few exceptions as in Québec, only our universities train nurses, and there is, of course, a Bachelor of Nursing, a Master of Nursing and a Doctor of Nursing; the last degree having curious semantics. Later in the text, we will talk about the "Nurse of Doctoring", the nurse practitioner.

Also, we saw the evolution of the registered nursing assistant. The RNA was to help the RN and BN with duties around the hospital floor, the emergency room, the delivery suite and so on. They were trained to complement the nursing team. They are now, for the most part, trained in community colleges and called Licensed Practical Nurses.

Several decades ago, nurses were trained to implement medical orders and to be at or near the patient's bedside round-the-clock. They provided continuous "nursing" and were the early-warning patient-monitoring system for the medical team.

Today's nurses are scientists with four-year science degrees. Today's nurses would prefer to be on the therapeutic multidisciplinary team and occupy some rungs on the therapeutic ladder. They want to be decision makers, and indeed this is now happening very rapidly for a variety of reasons.

The improvement in the quality and training of the

Canadian nurse has far outstripped nurses' positioning on the human resource team, the therapeutic ladder in the health system. **The Canadian nurse, like all our health providers, is one of the best prepared educationally and clinically in the world.** They are of high quality and integrity, full of compassion and of high and uniform quality compared to other developed countries. The OECD (Organization for Economic Co-operation and Development) countries have approximately six nurses per thousand population, and Canada has about eleven per thousand Canadians. This is an adequate supply of nurses, but unfortunately, they are grossly mis-applied in the system creating the impression of undersupply.

As well, we have an impending wave of nursing retirements approaching rapidly, that we have not dealt with adequately. This is paramountly similar to the situation with family medicine and specialty medicine.

In the past twenty years or so, the nursing profession has grappled with the health system to re-design and re-structure their participation. Nurses want their profession to be recognized, valued and accepted for what they do and can do.

Many of the reasons for the rather slow evolution of the nursing profession have been the result of an inability to adapt to changing conditions because of hospital administration rules that have stifled innovation and promoted inflexibility.

Hospital Administration rules and procedures, along with liability issues, to a large degree have pre-

vented and obstructed the progress of the nursing profession.

Much of this element of inflexibility and inability to change and adapt has been caused by the profession's own fear of liability. Thirty years ago, there was oftentimes more flexibility based on the integrity and experience of the individual nurse in the local system. It was not unusual for a nurse with considerable emergency room experience but less formal training than today, at four in the morning to order an x-ray of a fractured leg. She would give some analgesic, straighten the leg, check the pulse and call the MD at eight a.m. This would certainly not happen in today's nursing world.

Clearly, evolution of the system has not allowed for evolution of the nurse's role in the system. When nurses who are eligible to retire today began their careers, they could not have gone to work without their mercury thermometers. Today they can forget the thermometers but had better not go to work without a pen. Paper work is voluminous and compulsory. It has pulled, if not ripped, the nurse away from the bedside and relocated her or him to the desk, and now, of course, to the computer terminal.

As nurses know, ward clerk duties now frequently fall mostly to the nurse. Ward clerks are personnel who do the clerical duties of a hospital ward or Emergency Department to allow the nurses to apply full attention to patient care. But ward clerks are mostly a thing of the past in order to cut costs.

As an MD I have often related humorously that it

would take one minute to give Mrs. Smith a bedpan and one minute to empty the contents. Mindlessly, however, it then takes ten to fifteen minutes for the nurse to write about the episode. This includes the time, color, shape, volume, texture and floaters or non-floaters. They even have to record what is not there: not black, no blood, no mucous and of course at the end, the usual "the patient tolerated the episode very well". Must follow procedures! One does not need a four-year science degree for that.

Fortunately, the system is correcting some of these issues; for example, charting by exception or charting only if the episode is outside the norm.

Nurses are now also expected to collect data in the system for all kinds of reasons. Probably a good thing for staffing efficiency, outcomes, and so on, but it is clearly at the expense of patient bedside care. Nurses have forms upon forms to fill, generally more than physicians and some-times for the physicians.

On one occasion I was at the supplies counter in our hospital. There was a staff person standing next to me with a form.

I asked for fun, "What do you have there?"

"It is a form."

"Form for what?" I responded.

"Oh, I need some forms."

Incredulously I said, "You mean you need a form to order forms?"

He answered, "Yes".

Is There a Shortage of Nurses?

Nurses now are highly-trained science-oriented health-care providers. *They should not be doing non-nursing duties that can easily be done by others with far less but adequate training.* **This factor alone if rectified would eliminate for the most part the alleged nursing shortage, and much professional discontent.**

You may have noticed I said *alleged nursing shortage*. Indeed, it is hard to rationalize the perennial public weeping and gnashing of teeth that is going on in the press in our country about various shortages. *Where in the western world are we short of anything?* Undoubtedly, the providers honestly and acrimoniously perpetrate and perpetuate this activity, but *our nursing numbers are some of the best in the world.*

One may ask then, What gives? How come? Where are they?

Are there really shortages? The answer is yes.

Are they specific? The answer is yes.

Are they global? The answer is no. They may become global, however, with impending retirements.

Will the shortage be solved by nurse practitioners? The answer is no.

Are there many nurses doing other sorts of non nursing jobs or not working at all? The answer is

yes.

Are nurses doing too much overtime? The answer is yes.

Will the problem be resolved only by training more nurses? The answer is no.

Will more training for some nurses solve the problem? The answer is yes, but only if we recognize their training and expertise in the appropriate way and if the collective agreements allow the process to occur.

Austerity in the system has encouraged having fewer nurses, most or all obliged to do lots of overtime and call backs, as opposed to adequate staffing with far fewer obligations beyond the forty-hour workweek, **because one and a half full-time-equivalent jobs done by one person generates only one set of benefits.**

This austerity also results in a high number of casual workers in the nursing system. But most nurses will not sit around for ten years as a casual employee with no benefits awaiting a full-time job. They want a job with benefits and security and not just casual work for forty hours a week. Without a permanent job and security, nurses cannot get mortgages, start families and get on with life!

Naturally, the more sophisticated and specialized the nursing job, the more difficult it is to abruptly replace the nurse. For example, it is virtually impossible to replace a nurse in our emergency rooms, cardiac care units, surgical intensive care units, operating rooms and so on. For these types of nursing jobs there is less likelihood, if any likelihood at all, that there will be any kind of replacement spontaneously available.

After all, we must remember that for the most part they are trained on the job. There is no pool of fully trained employees sitting around waiting for such fill-in work. Inevitably, the replacement can only be one of the other staff members who is asked to do extra duty to cover a colleague's illness, vacation, absence related to obligation to one's family or just plain burn-out, a modern day social or workplace diagnosis that seems not to fit anywhere medically.

I once heard it said by an administrator "a nurse is a nurse, they are all the same". Not so, any more than a lawyer is a lawyer, a doctor is a doctor, a teacher is a teacher, or a painter is a painter. A pilot is not a pilot either. Otherwise, with a general pilot's license one could fly an airliner. Small chance!

Rebuilding Human Resources

There are nurses with considerable ability and experience that cannot be replaced by another nurse.

We do not have enough nurses with higher clinical and academic training and experience in our system because we do not pay them proportionately. These are the nurses that do the highly specialized, intense, and difficult care. Oftentimes, there is no incentive beyond idealism and academic challenge to be one of these nurses. As a matter of fact, there are numerous disincentives, involving cost of training, lifestyle, workplace issues, and intensity of daily routine.

More entrants in nursing schools will not solve the problem any more than having more family doctors will give us more cardiac surgeons. Increased general production does not mean overflow will go to the areas of specific need.

We are back to square one again on health-human-resource planning. **What exactly are the shortages? Where are they? How are they weighted? Very importantly, how should the shortages be rectified?** Is it up to the schools of nursing to know what the needs of governments are on an ongoing basis?

A good friend of mine once said that if you go into a store and you do not know what you are looking for, chances are you won't find it!

And last but not least, the biggest dilemma, who will do it? **Who has the responsibility;** surely it is not the universities and their schools of nursing? Again we have the same problem: No communication between the widget maker and the widget user.

Who has the responsibility to manage health-human resources produced by independent academic institutions in a system governed by federal legislation when jurisdiction is totally in the hands of the provinces and territories, and operations are in the hands of regional health authorities?

The provinces and territories are in charge of their health systems. The Canada Health Act is federal legislation yielding mixed jurisdiction.

This provincial-territorial jurisdiction was decided by the founding fathers in 1867 and consolidated in the British North America Act. **The federal government now wants in on the control of health.**

"Aye! Now there's the rub." Anyone have any suggestions? Is health care a federal responsibility? Is it a provincial responsibility? Is it the responsibility of the universities? Who is accountable to whom? Alberta could easily soon tell the feds to keep their thirteen percent; that they will run their own health system with a new 'Alberta Health Act'.

It is startling that we continuously hear that the solution to the nursing shortage problem and the doctor shortage problem is categorically more entrants into the profession.

If the health system was not open-ended and not publicly funded, if the health system was totally private with users paying the doctors and nurses directly, I am sure the current numbers of doctors and nurses would somehow be adequate and there would be alternate suggestions. We never hear accountants, plumbers, lawyers, insurance agents or carpenters saying, "They do not have enough of us!" Only public servants seem to echo this refrain.

*Clearly in today's Canadian Health Care Sys-
tem, we have a colossal inappropriate and ineffective
use of all our human resources. We are delivering in
anno domini 2004 a product with an anno domini 1960
mentality and methodology, and sometimes people.
Soaring costs are partially attributable to this.*

Facing "Crisis"

**We have heard the word 'crisis' now for fifteen
years from the providers in the system. I believe it is
hardly a crisis in the true definition when it has continued for fifteen years.**

**Remember we are describing one of the best, if
not *the* best, system in the world.**

Last year I could only smile while listening to a rep-
resentative of one of our national professional medical organizations escalate a notch on the acrimony scale.
"Canada is experiencing a health care catastrophe!" Yikes!
What is next?

I suppose the word "crisis" does not gather much
attention anymore. In medicine we call this concept an-
ergy or tachyphylaxis. Alright guys, let's try cataclysm,
apocalypse, black hole, annihilation or ground zero, or
maybe a little more scientifically, maximum entropy. That
should convince everyone that the system is falling apart
and help shift more government money into the system.

**More money allocated to the health care sys-
tem now and proposed as an only solution to our prob-**

lems will surely weaken the system, not strengthen it, because we still will be ignoring the basic problems.

More money beyond annual inflationary growth will surely weaken the basic fiscal soundness of governance in Canada, federal, provincial and territorial, and subsequently therefore health care. **Did the extra money, fifteen billion or thereabout, that we put in over the past decade make a difference?**

Should some money inside the system be redistributed? You bet! Should money paid to doctors be redistributed more appropriately? You bet even more! High-level medical care is under-funded and simple rudimentary elementary care is often unnecessary and funded too well. High-level medical care is under-funded considerably in Canada. Invasive cardiology, cancer treatment, neurosurgery and some other disciplines are all in great demand and under-staffed and under-funded. Simple high volume medicine and surgery is being over-used and is readily accessible, and has dubious need and outcomes.

One morning on rounds, I entered a patient's room. There were two new nursing grads previously unknown to me in the room. Two beaming enthusiastic young faces undoubtedly with student loans, now happily making twenty dollars or more an hour. I introduced myself, said, "Welcome on board", and reviewed my patient, who was in a geri-chair. The two new grads were there throughout the patient visit busily and conscientiously making a bed! Be sure to get the corner right. Right! Not a great career start after four years of science training, I would suspect.

Recognizing a Job Well Done

Recognition of advanced nursing experience and expertise is virtually unknown in our health care system.

As stated above, in many provincial systems after only a few short years there is no more financial or promotional incentive for nurses to stay on, train or improve. Only intrinsic professional idealism moves nurses to academic and career improvement. Vertical incentives are not readily attainable or realistic enough to retain nurses in the system.

There are virtually no incentives for moving horizontally either. **Highly specialized nurses** in cardiac care units, neonatal intensive care units and neuro-surgical units **are more often than not paid the same as floor staff.** Further university training for the most part will not garner any more income. **For the most part, job advancement is relegated only to moving on to supervisory positions and jumping on the administration ladder.** *Invariably, both of these preclude bedside nursing.* One rarely sees supervisory personnel working with the bedside nursing staff; they are usually office-bound.

The structure and organization of the Canadian Health Care System that nurses endure creates the public acrimony that we hear these days very frequently from the profession and encourages professional dissatisfaction.

Nurses for the most part have patient responsibility and no concomitant authority. Again, this is propagated by the system's liability concerns, traditional medical mores, inflexible collective agreements and sundry other issues.

Today's nurse is doing far more sophisticated work than thirty years ago. In those days, nurses usually could not insert intravenous lines, could not read a cardiac rhythm, and did little clinical evaluation of patients beyond observation, personal care, delivery of medication and vital signs. Today's nurse is much more capable, more sophisticated and has relieved the doctors of many duties.

I remember a call when I was in training in medicine thirty years ago. It was four in the morning. The nurse-in-training was obviously new and asked me to go immediately to the ward. I answered, "Why?"

"I need to know if I should call a cardiac arrest!"

I went immediately. The patient had had a sleeping pill and had a good pulse.

This would not happen today.

Today's well-trained cardiac-care-unit or emergency-room nurse will frequently have diagnosed an acute heart attack or heart failure and started initial protocol treatment before the medical doctor arrives.

Nurses in this country have the highest incidence of lost time on the job due to injury of any profession.

Most of this lost time is related to back injury sustained while lifting patients. Inevitably, nurses are expected to lift patients twice or even three times their own weight. The toughest, hardest working labor men anywhere in society are not allowed or expected to do the same on a construction or worksite. What happened to male orderlies who are appropriately muscled?

Full Scope Nursing

Registered nursing assistants or licensed practical nurses now also want to be on the therapeutic ladder. They want to use their training to do some of the duties traditionally relegated only to registered nurses.

Everybody, including those in the allied health professions, such as physiotherapy, respiratory therapy, occupational therapy, pharmacy, speech-language pathology and ultrasound technology, has moved onto and up the therapeutic ladder.

Only the medical general practitioner has complacently come down the ladder, continues to be pushed off the lower rungs of the ladder by others and continues to occupy overall fewer rungs on the ladder.

Full scope nursing practice is needed now more than ever. Barriers to the concept should be removed with the appropriate clinical practice guidelines applied.

Approximately three quarters of the nurses in Canada do not have a university degree; they are registered nurses with a diploma. Therefore, one quarter have a degree, the Bachelor of Nursing. The latter component, the Bachelor degreed nurse, is increasing inversely with the diploma nurse as the profession advances, and at some point all nurses will have a degree, the Bachelor of Nursing. **Full scope nursing practice can and will have a large impact on the health system, more especially on the family doctor.**

Nurse practitioners, clearly not a new concept, are now being touted as a salvation for the health system's difficulties.

Nurse practitioners originally were given more clinical diagnostic training to be able to work in remote areas devoid of physicians. The original concept was developed for the Canadian far north regions. There was much area to cover where endless snow, other geographical problems and isolation had to be faced. The nurse practitioner would do hugely heroic medical and surgical things to save lives in tents, on planes and traveling on dog sleds. Humorously, they would deliver babies in canoes with one hand while fighting off polar bears with the other!

Nurse practitioners have been tacitly accepted and practically rejected by the medical establishment.

The nurse practitioner can best be described as a talented nurse who has gained, through experience, expert clinical diagnostic judgment and acumen.

These nurses are capable of performing a large number of the duties of a family doctor. This expertise is clearly best gathered through substantive clinical-practice experience and not more academic training devoid of experience, lest they be educated beyond their practical clinical ability.

The concept of allowing and expanding full scope practice for all nurses in the system rather than promoting nurse practitioneering for a few nurses will have a huge impact on the service needs in the health system. Certainly full scope practice for all general nurses will have more impact than nurse practitioners who need advanced-training Masters degrees as they are now conceptualized. These impressions are currently playing out across the country as many nurse practitioners with advanced training are without jobs.

What Now?

So where do we go with nursing? The profession's leaders continuously say that care is inadequate because of nursing shortages. Yet if one asks about the quality of individual nursing care, they say it is excellent. I think it is excellent as well, but it needs change. I heard a national leader of the profession once say vehemently at a high level meeting in the presence of the Federal Minister of Health, that Canada's health care system was "worse than in the third world". This person obviously had not seen the "third" world. It was clearly an indefensible, emotional and ridiculous statement.

The nursing profession, in my estimation, needs to be redesigned and reformed as much as or more than primary medical care. Maybe both professions at the community-based level offer currently, in essence, the same challenge.

Change to reflect the modern circumstance is needed in the nursing and physician primary care workplace. A national plan that is not self-serving to the professions but that is rational for the system is clearly needed.

The health care system was put in place for the people of Canada. It was clearly put in place for the patients of Canada and not for the providers or pur-veyors, be they doctors, nurses, allied health profes-sionals, or politicians. The restructuring of health-human resources in the health system must suit only the valid consumers that the system must serve, not the providers. Then and only then will we get it right: Patient focus versus provider focus.

CHAPTER 7

Pharmacy

Chemical Therapeutics

In this chapter, I will attempt to reveal the huge and mostly positive changes that have taken place in health care as a result of the chemical therapeutic industry over the last forty years. These have been very positive changes that have been largely unappreciated by many consumers and providers alike.

There are over three hundred and thirty million prescriptions written a year in Canada. "Drugs" is the street name for both illicit and licit chemicals. We traditionally termed our chemical therapeutic outlets as "drug stores" or even more remotely, "the chemist" or "the apothecary". Today, they are more likely to be pharmacies with pharmacists, possibly in an effort to distance us from the word "drug" and the modern semantic connotation of the word. People today talk about taking their pills or medication as opposed to taking their drugs.

What is in a Name?

The research-based pharmaceutical industry has a difficult time these days to find names for new drugs. Indeed, the new chemical names are usually the most un-expected, unpronounceable and forgettable combinations of the twenty-six letters of the alphabet that one could ever conjure up. And unfortunately and ominously, almost every drug has two or more names.

Indeed, it is amusing to see how the meanings of words have changed. Grass, gay, hit, ecstasy, hash, queer, and weed have to be used with some caution today. When I was growing up in St. John's, it was quite usual to hear a humorous person being described as a 'queer hand'. Grass was something you mowed. Gay meant happy. Dope meant a person not too smart. Hit was a verb. Ecstasy was a desirable mood. Hash was yesterday's meat and potatoes. Queer meant odd. Dykes held back water. A weed was an unwanted plant. Now, in Canada, if you are introduced to a person and the question arises, "Are you married?" a yes answer must be followed by "To a man or a woman?" Things change.

Some years ago, one elderly female patient said to me, "Doctor, I don't know what I'm gonna do".
I responded: "What's the problem?"
"Well, Doctor, my old man is after me all the time."
Again, I responded: "What do you want me to do?"
"I heard there are some new pills out for that now. They're called 'Losex'! Could you give him some?"
"Not really. Those are for stomach problems, Missus."

"Oh, OK. His stomach is alright."

In the same vein, on another occasion, prior to more recent discoveries, an older lady said to me: "Doctor, are there any pills you can give my husband?"

I inquired: "What for? Is he sick?"

"No, Doctor, he can't... ya know... perform... ya know... it's been a long time... you know what I mean. I heard one of my girlfriends say the other day that since her husband is taking his new pills, he is much better in that department!"

"Oh? What's the name of the new pills?" I asked.

She responded, "Up Johns! It's written right on the pills."

"Well, Missus, I don't think those will work for your husband."

"That's fine, Doctor, you know best!"

A Pill for Everything

Chemical therapeutics are truly almost magical today. Indeed society thinks that there is a pill for everything. Fifteen billion dollars worth or more this past year, up fifteen percent per year and just about fifteen percent of all costs of health care. Coughs, colds, boils and sore moles; pimples on parts unspeakable, for all ailments self-inflicted and of decades duration; either the pink ones, the small ones, the big ones, the blue ones, the square ones, the round ones, the capsules, the elixir; the gum or the patch... There is something for it!

Patient: "There's gotta be something for 'that' today, Doctor. Sure we have a man on the moon!"

The doctor would muse, "How many times have I heard that?"

Doctor: "I'm sorry, Mr. Patient, we don't have anything for 'that' yet!"

Patient: "Well then, can I see a specialist?"

Doctor: "You really don't need to."

Doctor (to himself): "Good candidate for a placebo."

Doctor: "OK, we'll make a referral to the specialist."

Some time later...

Patient: "I saw that specialist you sent me to, Doctor. He was very good, ya know... knows his stuff... told me the same thing you did."

Doctor: "I'm glad. What can I do for you today?"

Patient: "Well, I came in to ask you, when something new comes out for 'that', Doc, would you give me a call?"

Doctor: "Sure, right away."

People take anything and everything today for every sort of reason. Medication is the fastest growing component of health care. Medication to get bigger if you are small, to get smaller if you are big; to grow hair, to remove hair; to sleep, to stay awake; to tan, to not tan; to go if you cannot, to not go if you go a lot; to have children, to not have children; to feel high if you are low, to feel low if you are high; to feel young if you are old, to feel old if you are young.

"They gotta have something for 'that' today, Doc. Sure we gotta man on the moon!" Darn Neil Armstrong anyway. One giant step for mankind and a continual hassle for MD's!

Thirty years ago, most physicians needed to know very well just a couple of dozen drugs to practice medicine. A physician had to know most of the adverse interactions and contraindications, and most physicians did know. Today, of course, there are as many families of drugs as there were routine drugs thirty years ago. It is impossible to know them all today and more difficult to know some of them well.

The pharmacist's computer is now the only method we have with any amount of reliability to prevent adverse interactions and allergic responses. Also, the pharmacist's computer is the only common denominator for surveillance in a world of polypharmacy, nominal duality as mentioned, doctor shopping, medication overuse, and over-the-counter drug misuse and abuse. Some drugs today cost more for an annual supply than doctors earned forty years ago.

Pharmacists are now also health educators. They provide instruction at the script counter that is invaluable. Traditionally, this instruction was provided by the doctor or the nurse; today it is provided very sparingly by them, if at all. Pharmacists also serve in hospitals today. Unusual thirty years ago, they now are an excellent and indispensable adjunct to patient care.

A patient once was reputed to have said to the doctor: "Doctor, those 'depositories' you gave me didn't work at all and they were terrible! For all the good they did me, I might as well have shoved them you know where!"

Patients need to have clear instructions on taking

their drugs. Many patients have large numbers of drugs, sometimes one drug because you are taking another. I call it the Burl Ives Syndrome. As his song goes, "She swallowed the spider to catch the fly... She swallowed the bird to catch the spider, etc..."

Some patients are instructed to take pills twice a day, some every twelve hours; some three times a day, some every eight hours; some four times a day, some every six hours; before meals, after meals; with food, without food; some go down the hatch, some go up another; some go on the skin, some go in the skin: Confusing? You bet, and that does not take into account poor vision or remembering to take them in the first place! Today the pharmacist has handily sorted out the great part of this patient quandary and medical risk.

The Benefits of Drugs

In my opinion, the sector of patient care that has advanced the most in the last thirty years is chemical therapeutics.

Chemical therapeutics is followed closely by the resoundingly improved investigative tools of today. Our laboratory and diagnostic imaging technology is excellent but our progress in chemical therapeutics has been unparalleled. New selective "target" drugs have changed forever the face and practice of medicine.

I vividly remember in the nineteen seventies walking the emergency room floor in our small rural hospital, all night on many occasions, with a number of severe childhood asthmatics. I would carry a syringe full of long acting adrenalin called "susphrine" in one hand and a child in the other. The child would be waxing and waning from pink to blue depending on intermittent doses of the syringe for life. It was all we had, along with oxygen and intravenous theophylline, to be used when treating children who were causing great concern on the part of the physician.

Today the asthmatic medications are immeasurably ahead of those days. Again, they are targeted to the offending organ tissue and its system. These drugs are good for the patient's breathing and the doctor's "nerves"!

A dear old doctor friend of mine, one of my mentors as a young physician, used to joke about a preparation available some forty years ago. It was apparently named "pheno-active". It was Phenobarbital and a laxative combo pill, an interesting combination of drugs to induce tranquilization and defecation; a tranquil biological experience every day. Medication has come, or should I say gone, a long way since "pheno-active".

I heard an internist describe to a patient once what he did as a specialist. He told the patient he was the same as a surgeon but he used pills instead of a scalpel to get people better. Interesting, curious and probably accurate.

Thirty-five years ago, for instance, the operating rooms of the country were full every morning with surgery for peptic ulcer disease. Stomach surgery was the bread and butter of general surgery. Now it is all but completely gone as a result of powerful acid-reduction blocking agents. Moreover recently, anti-bacterial treatment for stomach infection causing ulcers has shifted even more work from the scalpel to the pill. A huge positive impact has been made on general surgery as we knew it and on productivity in society by chemical therapeutics.

Anti-anginal drugs and thombolytics, or clot removing drugs, both given for acute heart attacks, stable angina and emergency unstable chest pains, are now so good that doctors are expected to stop heart attacks in progress and even reverse the process in just a few hours! Soon the same will be true for strokes.

A patient once said to me while I was taking a family history that her father had died of a "celebrated hemorrhage of the brain", a cerebral hemorrhage. During my training, I asked another patient what her father died of. She responded: "He died of a Sunday morning." A Newfoundland response! Patient education has come a long way.

Chemical therapeutic agents have emptied our mental institutions. Existing community-based services or de-institutionalization for the mentally ill and mentally challenged could never have occurred to the current degree over the last twenty years without the significant strides that have been made with psychotropic drugs.

Also, about sixty percent of all cancers are now cured, through many therapies, but largely because of new powerful chemical anti-cancer agents used in concert with surgery and radiation treatments.

Medications for blood pressure control are excellent today and have significantly reduced the incidence of acute cerebral strokes, brain injury and death. Possibly this factor has augmented the number of "residual" patients appearing now with chronic kidney failure, a slower more insidious onset process secondary to the adverse effects of blood pressure.

New medications generally also have fewer adverse side effects and are far better absorbed through the intestines.

The Cost

During 2002, it appears that expenditures on chemical therapeutics in Canada for the first time exceeded expenditures on physician services; a number somewhere over fifteen billion dollars.

We are now experiencing DTCA (direct to consumer advertising), usually on television. This bold approach is more typical of the American system and is encouraging the "pill generation" to increased consumption. At the turn of the century and millennium, Canadians spend approximately $400 per capita. Americans spend approximately $700 US per capita, and Egyptians spend approximately $15 US per capita.

North Americans spend mostly on anti-ulcer drugs and lipid-lowering drugs. Egyptians spend mostly on antibiotics.

The Japanese spend about $400 US per capita, mostly on lipid-lowering drugs and anti-ulcer drugs.

Recently, we have seen direct-to-consumer genetic tests marketed for cancer risk determination. I feel this is adding risk to the patient. It may be better to have a cancer and deal with it than to worry all one's life about getting one. The genetic testing may determine that the patient has a higher risk of contracting a certain cancer over a lifetime, but what does one do then? These things should be left to the discretion of the medical profession. Genetic profiling of patients, however, is now a bold new pharmaceutical frontier.

Most provinces have prescription drug programs to supply chemical therapeutics to those patients who cannot afford them. These programs are continually lambasted and berated by the medical community. This is in spite of the fact that physicians for the most part, along with pharmacists, make up the decision-making committees. Bureaucrats only carry out the program by the rules.

What could the doctors of Canada do for their poor and elderly patients if there were no government prescription drug programs, no way to treat these patients? The written prescription would be functionally useless. **The disease would be untreated. Government run prescription drug programs are excellent.**

I estimate that about seven billion dollars a year is spent cumulatively on the government prescription drug programs (PDP) across Canada. The global **costs are doubling about every four to five years. Physicians have to appreciate and realize that uncontrolled writ-**

ing and filling of prescription drug program scripts with no accountability or cost control will rapidly lead to program collapse. The very best diagnosis is functionally useless without therapy.

Who Pays?

There is no bucket of money or pot of gold for health spending in the capital cities of Canada, including Ottawa. Simplistically, the money for prescription drugs has to come from somewhere. The first step in eliminating public debt is obviously to stop adding to it. It means we must balance government budgets continuously and live within our means. Only this concept of fiscal soundness and responsibility will secure the future of public health care for those who are truly ill, and guarantee sustainability. The federal debt is now about twenty thousand dollars per capita. Provincial debts are mostly about half of this amount! Social development cannot precede economic development.

Physicians and patients, by and large, do not give even a second thought to costs, either for prescriptions or other. It is free, right? The government is paying.

Astoundingly, governments do not know individual costs of a service either! The most expensive treatment is therefore often thought to be the best. Of course patients almost universally think that health care is free. They pay taxes and therefore they feel they have the inalienable right to consume any amount they want of the most expensive care or therapy, whether they need it or not.

Overuse of prescription drugs is analogous to the auto-mobile insurance difficulties that now exist in Canada, fraught with the human factor over personal injury claim abuse.

Will putting more money blindly into our publicly funded health care system remotely change any of this human behavior? My opinion is that it most definitely will not. Not for either the providers or the consumers.

The recent Romanow Report recommended allo-cation of additional new money. This money negotiated by the Premiers with Ottawa will disappear with a large and loud-but-short sucking noise. The federal government is now backing off on its commitment, citing the provinces and territories have not lived up to their end. There will be an even shorter sucking noise!

Sixty-five percent of health care costs are consumed by salaries paid to workers in the system. Conceptually then where do we put the Kirby and Romanow Reports that suggest five billion more dollars a year to be allocated, again probably sixty-five percent to providers? Have we really defined the problem? I think not. As yet, there is too much denial and too much avoidance of voter ire. Noth-ing is being done to address the patient demand side. Nothing is being planned for the patient demand side. We continue to cut a foot off the bottom of our blanket and sew it on the top to make it longer.

Pharmacy is probably a better buy in Canada than many physician services or hospital services. Simply put, this is because the fundamentals of insurance are only somewhat present in pharmacy in Canada relative to other health services. And for the most part, in pharmacy there is a patient co-pay, a deductible, or patient participation in costs. Patients complain about this vehemently because it is supposed to be free, right? After all, it is health.

Cross-Border Shopping

Pharmacy is much cheaper in Canada than in the United States for various reasons. Hence we are seeing the evolving mail order cyber pharmacy.

Cyber pharmacy or cross-border prescribing by Canadian physicians for unseen and unknown patients in the United States is wrong.

Cross-border prescribing is a paramount manifestation of the differences between the Canadian egalitarian approach to health care and the American capitalistic approach.

Canadians have historically controlled drug costs with legislation. Let the American legislators do the same for their citizens.

Canadian physicians who participate in this activity should be sternly warned by our license and discipline authorities, our Colleges of Physicians and Surgeons, to cease and desist immediately or their licenses will be removed.

Physicians who sell their signature for distant unknown and unseen patients' treatments are breaking an ancient creed of the medical profession.

Applying Insurance Principles

The basic fundamental principle of any insurance plan does not exist in Medicare's funding of physicians' services or hospitalization, and this is not for any good reason. Then what will or can control utilization? Should we continue to try to take care of everything that comes in the health door? Obviously, the only cost control factor in our system today is the maximized volume of activity the system is capable of flowing through, the so-called "soft cap" on services. However, some volume control determinants have been applied by governments to some of the providers. Many provinces for instance, have salary caps on physicians.

Some advocates have suggested that we Canadians should start a national pharmacare program, most notably, the National Health Care Forum of the mid-nineties and now Mr. Romanow's report. **I believe it is possible to design a national pharmacare program if the fundamentals are right and there is prorated patient participation in costs with inherent catastrophic cost protection provision.** Otherwise, it will be a certain spending hemorrhage and a short lifespan likened to piercing one's aorta.

Health Canada's Health Protection Branch must expedite and expand its assessment and certification of new drugs. It is not good enough to ignore and not somehow rate the efficacy of new drugs. It is not good enough to ignore and not somehow rate cost-benefit analysis. It is not good enough to ignore and not rate somehow quality-adjusted life-years of new medications.

Currently, drugs are assessed only for adversity. In other words, "We have tested this drug. If you take it for whatever it is said to be designed for and as prescribed, it will not kill you!" The Canadian Standards Association (CSA) does a markedly better job of assessing the quality and safety of manufactured products. Health Canada also needs to overhaul the system that monitors drugs after they are put on the market. Adverse drug reaction monitoring will save lives.

What Lies Ahead?

We can look forward in the future to more and more sophistication and benefit from chemical therapeutics along with more and more sophistication of health care and cost challenges. In this country and America, we are close to having available mechanical hearts, totally implantable devices of considerable cost along with the many implantation devices we have available now. There are large numbers of patients with the need and indication. As people say, "Soon enough, there will be something for 'that'."

It is interesting that in the past several years the federal government has itself unwisely embarked on its own into the world of pharmacy, or should I say drugs. They somehow found or picked something for 'that'. They should stick to governance and stay out of the science of chemical therapeutics. I am of course 'reeferring' to medical marijuana. Now they want to pilot a program of selling marijuana in pharmacies. All pharmacies should refuse. Smoking a green leaf, whether it is tobacco or marijuana, has the same risk for dangerous disease. The federal government should stop this immediately.

The federal government should know that marijuana is not one of those "somethings" mentioned above. **There is no such thing as medical marijuana.** Medical marijuana is a medical myth, **so much bovine excrement**, conjured up by the federal government for whatever inconceivable reason.

CHAPTER 8

Older People and Long-Term Care

Long-term institutional care has two divisions. The first one is continuing care for those fragile individuals of any age who are too ill or disabled to reside in the community even with support services. The second division, by definition, is for those individuals who are not ill but who are too old, frail, insecure, and alone to live at home. Therefore, they need the security of communal institutional living with supervision.

Home care, in contrast to both groups mentioned above, is designed somewhat differently in that it is obviously delivered in the patient's home. Part or full time providers go to the consumer-patient's home to give care. It may be of varied and adjustable intensity and usually leads eventually to institutional care.

Family Patterns

Previous to the availability of these social systems, our elderly usually lived with their families or lived perilously alone with community or neighborhood supervision. Traditionally, homes usually had a continuous presence, inevitably female. Three-generation households used to be the norm. The father eventually became the son and the mother eventually became the daughter. Households changed from two generations to three generations, back to two and on to three again. Sometimes there were four generations. It was the cycle of life, the family.

The family represented one's long-term security, not the government. Today, households are, for the most part, only one or two generations. The need and desire for two providers in the modern family has changed things. Homes are now, for the most part, empty during daytime. This phenomenon has led to the need for daycare and pre-schools for our progeny and non-family based end-of-life care.

Seniors are living longer and better lives today. Also, they prefer and demand independence as long as possible. **The average age of entry to nursing homes throughout Canada today is eighty years plus.**

When Medicare was introduced forty years ago, a working life usually started at twenty years of age and ended at sixty-five or more. There was no freedom fifty-five; it was arrival at sixty-five and a rocking chair purchase. Providers usually spent forty-five years in the work force and ten years or less in retirement. The actuarial numbers fit the needs of the collective societal demands.

Today, our working lives start at twenty-five years of age at the earliest and are usually expected to finish at "freedom" fifty-five. Approximately thirty years of work life and twenty-five years of retirement.

The actuarial numbers do not fit. We are living now to eighty-two years of age or so on average. The productive portion of our lives is much less.

The global dependency on the current and shrinking working population is already great and getting greater. This is a major social quandary for this country and other developed countries. **How will we continue to fund our current social programs with more and more consumers and progressively fewer providers?**

How can we possibly think of adding another program? Pharmacare? Long-term care? Mr. Romanow has not explained where the funding would come from. He has suggested that we increase the supply of services to the aged and infirm but has again totally ignored the financial demand that it would incur.

In reality, too big a segment of our population will soon be living on pensions and government programs dependent upon resources yet to be generated by the working people. This direction seems to be rather ominous when we look at the imminent population bulge of elderly people, the baby boomers and the x-generation. Also ominous is the likelihood and almost certainty of a super-imposed wave of premature cardiovascular disease and diabetes in younger than usual age groups. The younger age groups are increasingly out of shape. "When I was your age, sonny, I had to get up and walk… to change the television channel!"

The Boomer Bulge

At the beginning of the peak load of the population of baby boomers, around 2014, we can expect two or three times the current number of age-related diseases and consequent societal needs. It will taper then to 2030 or thereabouts, when the funeral home industry, the last people to let us down, will have happily dealt with most of the postwar baby boomers. They have even figured a way to get the boomers' money sooner, pre-pay. Pay now, be buried or cremated later.

In the meantime, we are not prepared in our acute health care system for the approaching baby boomers, nor are we ready in the long-term care system for them. Mr. Romanow has suggested in his recommendations more funding and extension of the Canada Health Act to include home mental health, home post-acute care and home palliative care. Recommendation thirty-four.

In effect, New Brunswick has the only prototype home-care system in place now. The Extra-Mural Program, a wonderful success and a tribute to Dr. Gordon Ferguson and all the employees, the 'Extra Mural Program' in New Brunswick is hospital service given in people's homes. Nurses, physiotherapists, social workers, and psychologists deliver hospital services in patients' homes.

In the acute care system, or the Canadian hospital system, we are not ready nor are we even preparing for the boomers.

We are able to surmise that in ten years we will have two to three age-related health episodes where today we have one! Age-related cancers, fractures, renal dialysis, cardiac events and so on will increase two to three fold. The extra human resources we will need for the hospital-based system ten years from now should be training now, and they are not. We cannot produce a cardiologist or the like in less than ten years.

One could also postulate with the same line of thinking, that under the current guidelines and practices for acute care we will need, in 2014, two to three hospital beds where we now have one! *That will not happen.* **But 2014 will see the early peak baby boomer health care load. The thin edge of this boomer wedge is starting now as I write and you read.**

Should we install double bunks? Yes, of course! That's the answer, double bunks! Hospital beds with two shifts of staff, one tall, and one short. Now that's a two-tiered health care system!

All humour aside, we are not even thinking of preparing for this huge health care consumption period. **A large part of this projected acute care need will have to be delivered at home in the patient's bed, the only bed that will be available**, I am sure. Mr. Romanow has that one right, but he makes no suggestions.

Logically, if our flow-through of patients today, volumization, is restricted or "hour-glassed" only by the volume and the availability of human resources as discussed above, how will we manage to flow through two to three times the volume very soon?

We cannot control the growth of social programs like health by only limiting dollars and not concomitantly limiting utilization and reducing comprehensiveness.

Our cardiac care system and our cancer care system, the two largest ones, will be woefully unable to pass the load of baby boomer patients through. Machinery, real estate and technology will not be the problem. They are easily had. **Specialist doctors, specialist nurses, allied health providers, and technicians will be the critical limiting factor** in those rapidly approaching and looming times of large demand and high expectations. **We are not ready.** Mr. Romanow seems not to have appreciated this fact. Everyone appears to be stuck in the present tense; tomorrow or the future tense seems to have been forgotten. Political future of course, never goes past five years federally and four years provincially.

The future need of specialist physicians, oftentimes called "real" doctors by some, is huge. On the other hand, as discussed, the general family doctor is moving towards self-imposed obsolescence. Many are doing only relatively simple "runny nose" medicine in large urban areas that represent sixty or seventy percent of Canada's population. Unimportant work makes the worker unimportant. Some family doctors make substantially more money than some specialists and are doing substantially less complicated medicine crammed into a smaller workweek. Much of this family doctor work, if not done at all, would make little or no difference at all.

Clearly, the short cut to managing the baby boomers' medical needs in the future is to encourage and direct as many young general practitioners as possible into the needed specialties and as soon as possible. And direct access to specialist care may be an improvement and may save resources. It needs to be studied.

Hospital Home Care

The baby boomers, quite ironically, have been used to having virtually all they wanted all their lives. Now they may not have their terminal health care well provided for even though they have ample money to pay for the best. This is another pressure that is pushing us towards duality.

Community or home-based acute care now must be urgently pondered and developed. Acute medical care that traditionally needed hospital admission will soon be sent back to the patient's own bed along with the appropriate itinerant health service staff and equipment.

Of course, these patients will need care at home provided by mobile acute health care teams with portable equipment. This model, as stated above, exists now in New Brunswick. It is called the Extra-Mural Program. The hospital with no walls. It has a wonderful reputation.

Extra-Mural nurses now do sub-acute and palliative care. They also do chronic care and post-operative care in this system. The model needs further evolution for the country. Nurses, who in essence are nurse practitioners, deliver all of this care in the home. Again, as stated earlier, **we do not have the human resources now or in our projections to completely accomplish this objective.** If we do not move rapidly on this plan, or any plan, soon, it will be a more than troublesome time for everybody: providers, patients and governments alike, in the next two decades.

Considering long-term care as a basic Canadian social principal and a universal program, we must, as a country, appreciate that the state cannot take care of every citizen's parents. We must take the responsibility individually for our elderly parents. The state can help, but the state cannot remotely consider doing everything. Mr. Romanow is raising expectations by suggesting this without any concern for raising money and therefore taxes.

Financial resources applied by the state to care for the poor elderly and the elderly needing costly custodial care are resented by some. Many families with the financial resources are obliged to care for their elderly. Many of these families, as a result of our social programs, also do not feel it is their responsibility. Many children want their parents' financial resources to flow to them and for government to care for their parents. Many parents feel the same. "We deserve it, Doc. We paid taxes all our lives! Those who never worked all their lives get it free."

End-of-parental-life "financial gymnastics" done by many children of seniors is tantamount to "deadbeat" offspring who have abandoned their parents. There is some irony in this phenomenon, which is now commonplace. Mom and Dad's money should take care of Mom and Dad in their old age; anything left over after death should go to the relatives. Many children of aging and unwell parents encourage and pressure their parents to divest their assets to their children as early as possible. The objective is to prevent government from "getting it".

Government should contribute only when the individual's resources have run out. Unfortunately, for some Canadians the mindset is different. They think it is the government's sole responsibility to take care of Mom and Dad.

Government money in support of any long-term senior care, as a rule should flow through to the client or legal guardian and not to the institution. This will contribute to accountability in long-term custodial care on the part of the private institutions and give alternate choices to the seniors and their families. Children of baby boomers will do well on inheritance in the next thirty years. The baby boomers are rich! Governments will do well also, as capital gains are triggered by the inheritance of baby boomers' properties by their beneficiaries.

CHAPTER 9

Health Care Myths

1.   Health care is free
2.   More spending equals better health care
3.   There is a family doctor shortage
4.   Antibiotics are always good things
5.   There is a nursing shortage
6.   Health care is under-funded
7.   Wellness equals the absence of illness
8.   There is a medication for everything
9.   Doctors rush because there are not enough of them
10. One must see a doctor if sick
11. Nurses cannot do doctors' work
12. General practitioners cannot do specialists' work
13. Licensed practical nurses cannot do nurses' work
14. More family doctors equals fewer people without one
15. Doctors do not make mistakes
16. Government is responsible for the individual's health
17. Administrative costs of health care are high in Canada
18. Hospital beds equal good community health care
19. All symptoms of illness are diagnosable

20.   All illnesses can be treated and cured
21.   More food equals better health
22.   Urban family doctors are better than rural family doctors
23.   It is somebody's fault if things do not go well medically
24.   Doctors' associations' complaints about the system are true
25.   Patient participation in costs of health care equals two tiers
26.   The system is in crisis
27.   Waiting means the system is bad
28.   Health education can be done in the health system
29.   A ten, twenty or thirty bed hospital is a hospital
30.   Nurse practitioners will solve the primary care problem
31.   All doctor visits are justified
32.   Private medical care in a public system equals two tiers
33.   Marijuana has medicinal properties
34.   The federal government takes good care of native health
35.   Everyone on a waiting list needs to be there
36.   Nurses unions' complaints about the system are true
37.   The health system cannot collapse
38.   Health is not all about money
39.   Departments of Health take care of health (not really, only illness)
40.   The federal department of health can take care of fitness
41.   More medical schools will solve doctor shortages
42.   The bigger the city, the better the health care

43.   An office visit equals one complaint

44.   Native health problems are health problems

45.   The health care system is sustainable

46.   Medical wants are medical needs

47.   The Romanow Report will help sustainability

48.   Patients paying for part of their health care is unacceptable

49.   We do not have two-tiered health care

50.   We are unable to fix health

CHAPTER 10

Recommendation

Health care in Canada is extremely large, important, and deserves much thought. I believe there are cardinal and basic structural problems on all three sides of
the health care triangle: patients, providers, and
governments, that make the system terminal. Logically,
then, any changes proposed for rectification have to be
made on all three sides of the triangle: the patient, the
provider, and the insurer.

**I have suggested that options for a prorated,
patient participation, tax-based system be developed.
Citizens who become patients should pay part of the
cost of their health care. There would be no user fees,
no cash seen anywhere, no obstruction to access to
quality health care, and clear protection for all patients
from catastrophic costs built directly into the system.**

This is the only possible way to have some inherent control on frivolous utilization and to combat the human factor for both consumers and providers. To be free
of cost is to be overused, misused and abused.

Sustainability, which means affordability, can only be had through this sort of process of utilization control and therefore cost control. There are many reasons why we should do this and few reasons why we should not. Then why not?

Accountability on all sides of the triangle should and would be achieved.

This whole question may be best answered by a national referendum, given that all else seems not to have given us a clear direction for our most valued and excellent health care system.

Let's fix it.

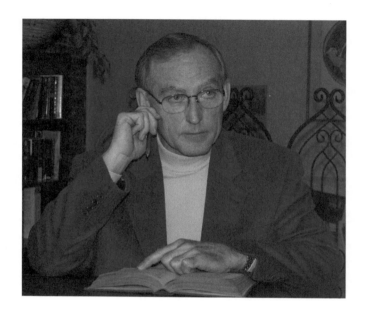

ABOUT THE AUTHOR

Dennis J. Furlong, MD, MSc, BMedSc, BPE has been a physician for thirty years, a general practitioner/family doctor in a rural practice in New Brunswick.

Preparation for his medical career began in his native Newfoundland at Memorial University, where he received his MD in 1976. Previously he had been a teacher trained in New Brunswick, where he received his Bachelor of Physical Education from UNB in 1967; and in Oregon, where he received his Masters degree at the University of Oregon in 1970 in the special education of children with learning disabilities.

From 1999-2003, Dr. Furlong was the MLA for Dalhousie-

East Restigouche (northern New Brunswick) in the first Lord government. He served two years as Minister of Education and two as Minister of Health.

Dr. Furlong is well known for his dedication to his profession, to his people, to the institutions of this country, and to the wider world, which he has served through amateur athletics.

He has served seven years on the Medical Council of Canada, sat as President of the New Brunswick Medical Society, President of the College of Physicians and Surgeons of New Brunswick, President of the New Brunswick Lung Association, President of the Premiers Council on the status of disabled persons of New Brunswick, Technical Director of the World Junior Track and Field Championships, and is a Rotary International Paul Harris fellow.

Dr. Furlong has three sons and three daughters-in-law and two grandchildren; Denny, Shelley and their daughter Jena of Moncton, Sean, Michelle and their daughter Hailey of Dalhousie and Robin and Dawn of Calgary.

Order Form

Medicare Myths
Dennis J. Furlong M.D.
ISBN: 1-894372-39-5
$24.95 CAN / $20.00 US

The following discounts apply for orders of 10 or more copies:
Bookstores and Retail Accounts: 40%+
Wholesalers: 46%+
Educational Institutions: 20%
Public Libraries: 20%
Medical practitioners/corporate clients: 40%

All orders must include applicable sales taxes.

Allow $3.00 S&H for single copies and $5.00 for multiple copies

Quantity	Unit Price	Amount
	$24.95 CAN	
	$20.00 US	
_____		_____
Applicable Discounts		_____
Applicable Sales Taxes		_____
Shipping and Handling		_____
TOTAL		_____

QUICKFAX or
e-mail your order:
Fax: (506) 632-4009
E-mail: dcpub@fundy.net

DreamCatcher Publishing
105 Prince William Street
Saint John, NB, Canada E2L 2B2
Web: www.dreamcatcherbooks.ca